AIR FRYER
COOKBOOK

Series 6

This Book Includes : "The Complete Air Fryer Cookbook + The Affordable Air Fryer Cookbook"

By Denise White

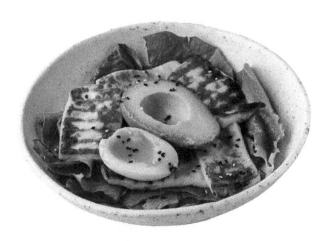

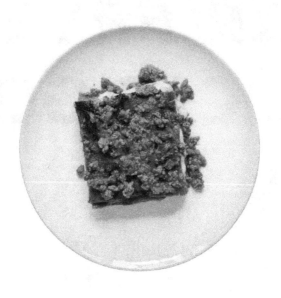

THE COMPLETE AIR FRYER COOKBOOK

Table of Contents

THE AFFORDABLE AIR FRYER COOKBOOK

Table of Contents

The Complete Air Fryer Cookbook

The Ultimate Cookbook With 100 Quick and Delicious Recipes for Quick and Easy Meals

By Marisa Smith

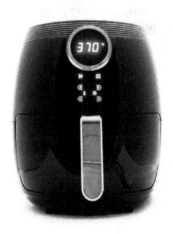

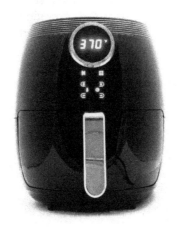

Introduction

Air fryers have seen a major increase in popularity, marketed as a healthy, guilt-free way to eat your favorite fried foods. These are believed to help increase the fat content of popular foods such as burgers, empanadas, chicken wings, and sticks of fish. But how good does an air fryer cook, exactly? The book will look at the facts to determine if many brands of air fryers do not need oil to work with the machine, but the taste of deep-fried food items can be improved by a few teaspoons. While air-fried food can be enjoyed with no oil, the benefit of the air fryer is that it only requires very little quantity.

Air Fryer Recipes

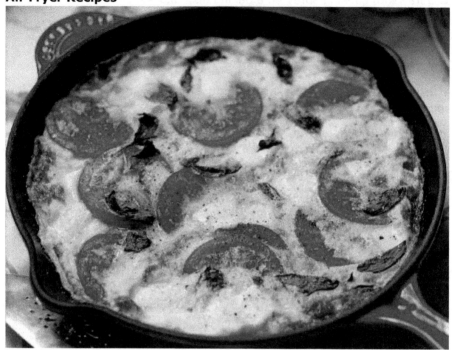

1.Basil Tomato Frittata

Total time: 35 min

Prep time: 15 min

Cook time: 20 min

Yield: 4 servings

Ingredients:

- 12 eggs
- 1/2 cup cheddar cheese, grated
- 1 1/2 cups cherry tomatoes, cut in half
- 1/2 cup fresh basil, chopped
- 1 cup baby spinach, chopped
- 1/2 cup yogurt
- Pepper
- Salt

Directions:

1. Spray with cooking spray on a baking dish and set aside.

2. Wire rack insertion at rack position 6. Pick bake, set temperature to 390 f, 35-minute timer. To preheat the oven, press start.

3. Whisk the eggs and yogurt together in a big bowl.

4. Layer a baking dish of spinach, lettuce, onions, and cheese. Pour the spinach mixture over the egg mixture, with pepper and salt, season.

5. Bake for 35 minutes in the oven.

6. Enjoy and serve.

2.Italian Breakfast Frittata

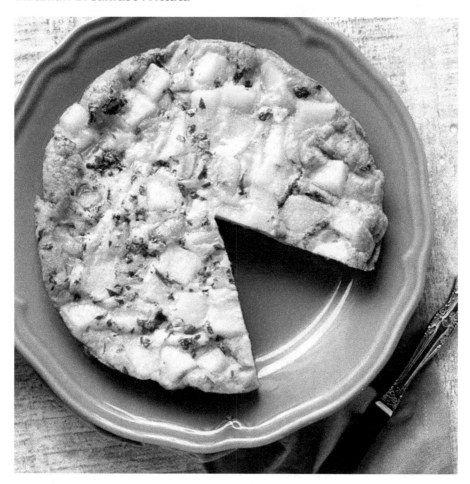

Total time: 35 min

Prep time: 15 min

Cook time: 20 min

Yield: 4 servings

Ingredients:

- Eight eggs
- 1 tbsp. fresh parsley, chopped
- 3 tbsp. parmesan cheese, grated

- Two small zucchinis, chopped and cooked
- 1/2 cup pancetta, chopped and cooked
- Pepper
- Salt

Directions:

1. Spray with cooking spray on a baking dish and set aside.

2. Wire rack insertion at rack position 6. Pick bake, set temperature to 350 f, 20-minute timer. To preheat the oven, press start.

3. Mix the eggs with pepper and salt in a mixing cup. Stir well and add parsley, cheese, zucchini, and pancetta.

4. Pour the egg mixture into the baking dish that has been prepared.

5. Bake a 20-minute frittata.

6. Enjoy and serve.

3.Healthy Baked Omelets

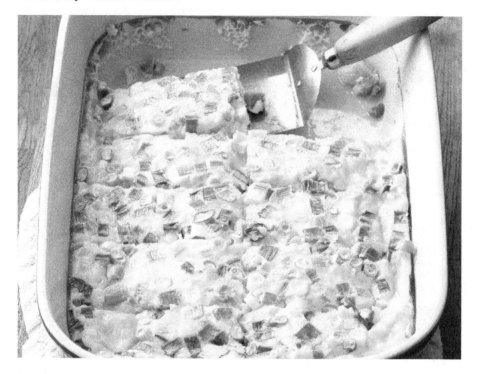

Total time: 45 min

Prep time: 10 minutes

Cooking time: 35 minutes

Yield: 6 servings

Ingredients:

- 8 eggs
- 1 cup bell pepper, chopped
- 1/2 cup onion, chopped
- 1/2 cup cheddar cheese, shredded
- 6 oz. ham, diced and cooked
- 1 cup milk
- Pepper
- Salt

Directions:

1. With cooking sauce, spray an 8-inch baking dish and put it aside.

2. Wire rack insertion at rack position 6. Pick bake, set temperature to 350 f, 45-minute timer. To preheat the oven, press start.

3. In a big cup, mix the milk, pepper, and salt with the eggs. Add the remaining ingredients and stir well.

4. Pour the egg mixture into the baking dish that has been prepared.

5. Bake for 45 minutes for an omelet.

6. Slicing and cooking.

7.

4.Easy Egg Casserole

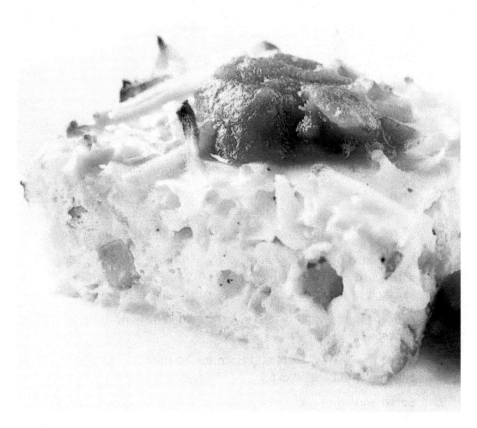

Total time: 55 min

Prep time: 10 min

Cook time: 45min

Yield: 8 servings

Ingredients:

- 8 eggs
- 1/2 tsp. garlic powder
- 2 cups cheddar cheese, shredded

- 1 cup milk

- 24 oz. frozen hash browns, thawed

- 1/2 onion, diced

- One red pepper, diced

- Four bacon slices, diced

- 1/2 lb. turkey breakfast sausage

- Pepper

- Salt

Directions:

1. Spray a 9*13-inch baking dish with cooking spray and set aside.

2. Insert wire rack in rack position 6. Select bake, set temperature 350 f, timer for 50 minutes. Press start to preheat the oven.

3. Cook breakfast sausage in a pan over medium heat until cooked through. Drain well and set aside.

4. Cook bacon in the same pan. Drain well and set aside.

5. In a mixing bowl, whisk eggs with milk, garlic powder, pepper, and salt. Add 1 cup cheese, hash browns, onion, red pepper, bacon, and sausage and stir well.

6. Pour the entire egg mixture into the baking dish. Sprinkle remaining cheese on top.

7. Cover the dish with foil and bake for 50 minutes. Remove foil and bake for 5 minutes more.

8. Serve and enjoy.

5.Flavor Packed Breakfast Casserole

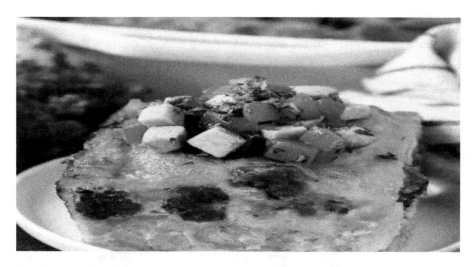

Total time: 50 min

Prep time: 10 minutes

Cook time: 40 minutes

Yield: 8 servings

Ingredients:

- 1 tsp. garlic powder
- 1 cup milk
- 12 eggs
- 1/2 cup cheddar cheese, shredded
- Two bell pepper, cubed
- 4 small potatoes, cubed
- 2 cups sausage, cooked and diced
- Pepper
- 1/4 cup onion, diced
- Salt

Directions:

1. With cooking oil, spray a 9*13-inch baking dish and put it aside.

2. Wire rack insertion at rack position 6. Pick bake, set temperature to 350 f, 40-minute timer. To preheat the oven, press start.

3. Add the cream, garlic powder, spice, and salt to the eggs in a big cup.

4. To the baking dish, add the bacon, bell peppers, and potatoes. Pour over the sausage mixture with the egg mixture. Sprinkle of onion and cheese.

5. Bake for 40 minutes in a casserole.

6. Slicing and cooking.

6.Vegetable Sausage Egg Bake

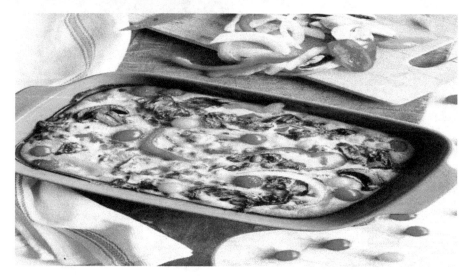

Total time: 45 min

Prep time: 10 minutes

Cook time: 35 minutes

Yield: 4 servings

Ingredients:

- Ten eggs
- 1 cup spinach, diced
- 1/2 cup almond milk
- Pepper
- 1 lb. sausage, cut into 1/2-inch pieces
- 1 cup onion, diced
- 1 cup pepper, diced
- 1 tsp. garlic powder

- Salt

Directions:

1. With cooking sauce, spray an 8*8-inch baking dish and put it aside.

2. Wire rack insertion at rack position 6. Pick bake, set temperature to 390 f, 35-minute timer. To preheat the oven, press start.

3. Whisk the eggs in a cup of milk and spices. Attach the sausage and vegetables and stir to mix.

4. Pour the egg mixture into the baking dish that has been prepared. For 35 minutes, roast.

5. Slicing and cooking.

7.Ham Egg Brunch Bake

Preparation time: 10 minutes

Cooking time: 60 minutes

Servings: 6

Ingredients:

- 4 eggs
- 20 oz. hash browns
- One onion, chopped
- 2 cups ham, chopped
- 3 cups cheddar cheese, shredded
- 1 cup sour cream
- 1 cup milk
- Pepper
- Salt

Directions:

1. Spray a 9*13-inch baking dish with cooking spray and set aside.

2. Insert wire rack in rack position 6. Select bake, set temperature 375 f, timer for 35 minutes. Press start to preheat the oven.

3. In a large mixing bowl, whisk eggs with sour cream, milk, pepper, and salt. Add 2 cups cheese and stir well.

4. Cook onion and ham in a medium pan until onion is softened.

5. Add hash brown to the pan and cook for 5 minutes.

6. Add onion ham mixture into the egg mixture and mix well.

7. Pour egg mixture into the prepared baking dish. Cover the dish with foil and bake for 35 minutes.

8. Remove foil and bake for 25 minutes more.

9. Slice and serve.

8.Cheese Broccoli Bake

Total time: 40 min

Prep time: 10 min

Cook time: 30 min

Yield: 12 servings

Ingredients:

- 12 eggs
- 1 1/2 cup cheddar cheese, shredded
- 2 cups broccoli florets, chopped
- 1 small onion, diced
- 1 cup milk
- Pepper
- Salt

Directions:

1. With cooking sauce, spray an 8*8-inch baking dish and put it aside.

2. Wire rack insertion at rack position 6. Pick bake, set temperature to 390 f, 35-minute timer. To preheat the oven, press start.

3. Whisk the eggs in a cup of milk and spices. Attach the sausage and vegetables and stir to mix.

4. Pour the egg mixture into the baking dish that has been prepared. For 35 minutes, roast.

5. Slicing and cooking.

9. Cheese Ham Omelets

Total time: 35 min

Prep time: 10 min

Cook time: 25 min

Yield: 6 servings

Ingredients:

- 8 eggs
- 1 cup ham, chopped
- 1 cup cheddar cheese, shredded
- 1/3 cup milk
- Pepper
- Salt

Directions:

1. With cooking oil, spray a 9*9-inch baking dish and put it aside.

2. Wire rack Insertion at rack position 6. Pick bake, set temperature to 390 f, 25-minute timer. To preheat the oven, press start.

3. In a big cup, mix the milk, pepper, and salt with the eggs. Stir in the cheese and ham.

4. In the prepared baking dish, add in the egg mixture and bake for 25 minutes.

5. Slicing and cooking.

9.Sweet Potato Frittata
Total time: 40 min

Prep time: 10 min

Cook time: 30 min

Yield: 6 servings

Ingredients:

- 10 eggs
- 1/4 cup goat cheese, crumbled
- 1 onion, diced
- 1 sweet potato, diced
- 2 cups broccoli, chopped
- 1 tbsp. olive oil

- Pepper
- Salt

Directions:

1. Spray with cooking spray on a baking dish and set aside.

2. Wire rack insertion at rack position 6. Pick bake, set temperature to 390 f, 20-minute timer. To preheat the oven, press start.

3. Heat oil over medium heat in a pan. Add the sweet potato, broccoli, and onion, then simmer for 10-15 minutes or until tender.

4. Mix the eggs with pepper and salt in a large mixing cup.

5. Cooked vegetables are moved to the baking dish. Pour over the vegetables with the egg mixture. Sprinkle with the goat's cheese and roast for 15-20 minutes.

6. Slicing and serving.

10.Toasty Grilled Chicken with Cauliflower and Garlic Butter

Total time: 45 min

Prep time: 10 min

Cook time: 35 min

Yield: 2 servings

Ingredients:

- Chicken legs
- 2 chicken legs (about 5 oz. each)
- ½ teaspoon garlic powder
- 1 tablespoon coconut oil
- ½ tablespoon Italian seasoning
- ¼ teaspoon salt
- Garlic butter
- 7 tablespoons unsalted butter, softened
- 2 garlic cloves, pressed
- 1 tablespoon fresh mint, finely chopped (optional)
- Salt and ground black pepper, to taste
- 10 oz. Cauliflower

Directions:

1. Mix the coconut oil and seasoning with the chicken wings.

2. For 60 minutes, set the air fryer to 350 degree F. You should flip it if it's 30 minutes out. They used forks and it was so simple.

3. Cut the florets of the cauliflower and cut the stem. Put to a boil in salty water in a saucepan for 5 minutes. To keep it warm, drain the water and put the lid on. Combine all the ingredients: a little bowl of garlic butter. Using cauliflower and garlic butter to serve the chicken.

11.Garlic Turkey

Total time: 30 min

Prep time: 10 min

Cook time: 20 min

Yield: 2 servings

Ingredients:

- 2 tablespoons coconut oil
- 2 lbs. turkey drumsticks
- Salt and pepper
- 1 lime, the juice
- 2 tablespoons avocado oil
- 7 garlic cloves, sliced
- ½ cup fresh basil, finely chopped

Directions:

1. Preheat up to 360 degrees Fahrenheit for your air fryer.
2. In an oil-greased baking pan, put the turkey bits. Salt and pepper with generosity.
3. Drizzle over the turkey bits with lime juice and avocado oil. Sprinkle on top of the garlic and parsley.
4. Air fried for 1 hour at 360 degrees Fahrenheit, spinning every 15 minutes or until the temperature within reaches 165 degrees Fahrenheit.

5.

12.Sweet and Sticky Turkey Wings

Total time: 30 min

Prep time: 10 min

Cook time: 20 min

Yield: 2 servings

Ingredients:

- 1 lb. turkey wings
- ½ teaspoon sea salt
- ¼ cup coconut amino
- ¼ teaspoon ginger minced
- 1teaspoon onion, chopped
- ¼ teaspoon garlic minced
- ¼ teaspoon chili flakes

Directions:

1. Preheat your air fryer to 360 degrees Fahrenheit.

2. Sprinkle fine sea salt on the wings

3. Air fry on 360 degrees Fahrenheit for 1 hour, turning every 15 minutes or until internal temperature has reached a temperature of 165 degrees Fahrenheit.

4. Heat a medium to a large skillet over medium heat, and add the coconut amino.

5. Add the minced ginger, minced garlic, chopped onion, and red pepper flakes (if desired). Once the sauce is simmering, start stirring. Keep stirring at regular intervals and adjust the heat as needed to keep cooking soft.

6. Once the sauce has thickened slightly, place the wings in a large heatproof bowl, and pour the sauce over them. Stir to coat and serve with sauce!

7.

13.Tofu and Cabbage Plate

Total time: 30 min

Prep time: 10 min

Cook time: 20 min

Yield: 2 servings

Ingredients:

- 1 cup tofu
- 7 oz. Fresh green cabbage
- ½ red onion
- 1 tablespoon coconut oil
- ½ cup Greek yogurt
- Salt and pepper

Directions:

1. To further extract excess liquid, push your tofu.
2. Split into squares or small bite-sized bits after pressing the tofu.
3. Bringing the air fryer into the basket.
4. Set the temperature to 370 degrees f. Please turn the air fryer on for 12 minutes.
5. Shred the cabbage and put it on a plate using a sharp knife or a mandolin.
6. Thinly slice the onion and add it to the pan, with the tofu and Greek yogurt added.
7. Drizzle the cabbage with coconut oil and apply some salt and pepper to taste.

14.Thai Fish

Total time: 30 min

Prep time: 10 min

Cook time: 20 min

Yield: 2 servings

Ingredients:

- ½ tablespoon coconut oil
- ¾ lbs. tuna, in pieces
- Salt and pepper
- 2 tablespoons olive oil
- 1 tablespoon green curry paste
- 7 oz. Canned, unsweetened coconut cream
- ½ cup fresh basil, chopped
- 1 lb. broccoli

Directions:

9. Put the pieces of fish into the baking tray. Generously salt and pepper and add a tablespoon of coconut oil to each piece of fish.

10. Combine the coconut cream, curry paste and chopped basil in a small bowl and pour over the fish.

11. Grease the bottom of the air fryer basket and place the fillets in the basket. Cook the steaks at 400 degrees for 10 minutes.

12. Meanwhile, cut the cauliflower into small florets and boil in lightly salted water for a few minutes. Serve with fish.

15.Chicken with Parsnips

Total time: 30 min

Prep time: 10 min

Cooking time: 20 min

Yield: 2 servings

Ingredients:

- 1 lb. chicken thighs or chicken drumsticks
- 1lb parsnips, peeled and cut into 2-3 inch pieces
- ½ tablespoon paprika powder
- Salt and pepper
- ¼ cup coconut oil
- ½ cup Greek yogurt
- ½ teaspoon garlic powder

- ½ teaspoon paprika powder
- Salt and pepper, to taste

Directions:

1. Preheat up to 360 degrees Fahrenheit for your air fryer.

2. In a baking pot, placed the chicken and the parsnips. Sprinkle with flour, paprika powder and pepper. Spray and coat generously with olive oil.

3. Fry the air for 1 hour at 360 degrees Fahrenheit, spinning every 15 minutes or until the temperature within exceeds 165 degrees Fahrenheit.

4. Mix the herb with the yogurt and eat along with the roasted chicken and parsnips.

16.Salmon Salad with Boiled Eggs

Total time: 30 min

Prep time: 10 min

Cook time: 20 min

Yield: 2 servings

Ingredients:

- 4 oz. Cucumber
- 2 spring onion
- 5 oz. Salmon
- ½ orange, zest and juice
- ½ cup Greek yogurt
- 1 teaspoon Dijon mustard
- 4 eggs
- 6 oz. Romaine lettuce
- 4 oz. Cherry tomatoes
- 2 tablespoons coconut oil
- Salt and pepper

Directions:

1. Finely chop the cucumber and the onion for the season. Place the salmon, orange, Greek yogurt and mustard in a medium dish. Remove to blend and season with salt and pepper. Only put aside.

2. In the basket, place the rack supplied with the fryer and place the eggs on the rack. Simply position it at the bottom of the air fryer basket if your air fryer does not have a grill. The temperature should be pressed at 250 and the time set at 15 minutes. Take them out and put them into the cool bathroom water to finish frying while the eggs are fried in the fryer. Break the eggs from the outer shell.

3. Place the salmon and egg mixture on a Romaine lettuce bed. Sprinkle with coconut oil and add the tomatoes. With salt and pepper, season.

17.Tomato Mint Soup

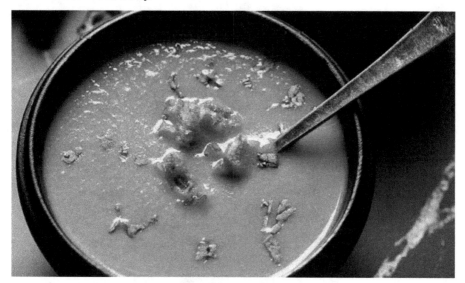

Prep time: 10 Minutes

Cook time: 20 Minutes

Yield: 2 servings

Ingredients:

- Oil for spraying
- ½ lb. red tomatoes cut in half
- 1 small red bell pepper quartered
- 1 small yellow onion quartered

- 1 small carrot chopped
- 4 garlic cloves peeled
- 1.5 cups water
- ½ cup coconut cream
- 4 fresh mint leaves finely chopped
- Grated goat cheese optional

Directions:

1. To keep it from sticking, brush the bottom of the basket with a bit of oil. In the air fryer, add the tomatoes, peppers, onions, carrots, garlic cloves and set to 360 degrees Fahrenheit and fry for 25 minutes.
2. In order to ensure an even roast, inspect the air fryer basket in half and shake it.
3. Place the vegetables in a medium-sized saucepan while the fryer is off, and apply the water to the pan. Let them cook the mixture. Decrease the flame and boil for 5 minutes or so. Mix the soup with the hand blender until finished, or let it cool and mix the soup with a conventional blender.
4. Add the coconut cream and mint. With salt and pepper, season. Goat cheese garnish.

18. Fried Cauliflower Rice

Prep time: 10 Minutes

Cook time: 20 Minutes

Servings: 2

Ingredients:

- 1 medium cauliflower
- 1 tablespoon coconut oil
- 3 spring onions, sliced
- 1 teaspoon smoked paprika
- 1/2 teaspoon ground cumin
- 1/4 teaspoon hot chili powder
- Salt

- Black pepper
- 50 g parmesan cheese, grated

Directions:

1. Remove and cut the cauliflower leaves into florets. Place the bomb in a food processor until it looks like rice.

2. Place the cauliflower rice with a little coconut oil in the air-fryer oven. Cook until lightly browned for 20 minutes, Scrape and apply chives, peppers, and seasonings from the sides of the air fryer cooker.

3. Let it cook for 10 more minutes, then add the cheese and let it cook for 5 more minutes. Re-scrape the sides of the oven and serve it with the ingredients of your choosing.

19.Baked Salmon

Total time: 15 min

Prep time: 05 min

Cook time: 10 min

Yield: 2 servings

Ingredients:

- 2 (6-oz.) Salmon fillets
- Kosher salt
- Freshly ground black pepper
- 2 teaspoons coconut oil
- 1 teaspoon garlic powder
- 1/2 teaspoon basil leaves

Directions:

13. Season the whole salmon with salt and pepper. Mix the coconut oil, garlic and basil in a small bowl. Spread on the salmon and place the salmon in the basket.

14. Set the fryer to 400 ° and cook for 10 minutes.

20.Prosciutto-Wrapped Parmesan Asparagus

Total time: 30 min

Prep time: 10 min

Cook time: 20 min

Yield: 4 servings

Ingredients:

- 1-pound of asparagus
- 12 (0.5-ounce) slices of prosciutto
- 1 tablespoon of coconut oil, melted
- 2 teaspoons of lemon juice
- 1/8 teaspoon of red pepper flakes
- 1/3 cup of grated Parmesan cheese
- 2 tablespoons of salted butter, melted

Directions:

1. On a clean work surface, place an asparagus spear on a slice of prosciutto.
2. Drizzle with lemon juice and coconut oil. Sprinkle the red pepper flakes and parmesan over the asparagus. A roll of prosciutto and an asparagus spear. In the Air Fryer, bring the basket in.
3. Set the temperature to 375 degrees F and set the timer for ten more minutes.
4. Sprinkle a roll of asparagus with butter before feeding. Enjoy!

21.Bacon-Wrapped Jalapeño Poppers

Total time: 30 min

Prep time: 10 min

Cook time: 20 min

Yield: 4 servings

Ingredients:

- 6 jalapeños (about 4" long each)
- 3-ounces of full-Fat: cream cheese
- 1/3 cup of shredded medium Cheddar cheese
- 1/4 teaspoon of garlic powder
- 12slices sugar-free bacon

Directions:

1. Break the tops off the jalapeños and slice down the center lengthwise in two parts. Break the white membrane and pepper seeds with care, using a knife.

2. In a large microwave-safe bowl, put the cream cheese, cheddar, and garlic powder. Remove from the microwave and stir for 30 seconds. Combine the jalapeños with a spoon of cheese.

3. Wrap about half of each jalapeño with a strip of bacon, covering the pepper completely. In the Air Fryer, bring the basket in.

4. Set the temperature to 400 degrees F and change the 12-minute timer.

5. Turn on the peppers halfway into the cooking stage. Serve it hot.

22.Garlic Parmesan Chicken Wings

Total time: 30 min

Prep time: 10 min

Cook time: 20 min

Yield: 4 servings

Ingredients:

- 2 pounds of raw chicken wings
- 1 teaspoon of pink Himalayan salt
- 1/2 teaspoon of garlic powder
- 1 tablespoon of baking powder
- 4 tablespoons of unsalted butter, melted
- 1/3 cup of grated Parmesan cheese
- 1/4 teaspoon of dried parsley

Directions:

1. Place the chicken wings, spice, and 1/2 teaspoon of garlic powder, baking powder, and toss in a large cup. Place the wings in the basket with the Air Fryer.

2. Change the temperature and set the timer to 400°F for 25 minutes.

3. During the cooking cycle, toss the basket two to three times.

4. Combine the sugar, parmesan, and parsley in a shallow dish.

5. Take the wings out of the fryer and put them in a large, clean dish. Over the wings, pour the butter mixture and toss until filled. Serve it hot.

23.Spicy Buffalo Chicken Dip

Total time: 30 min

Prep time: 10 min

Cook time: 20 min

Yield: 4 servings

Ingredients:

- 1 cup of cooked, diced chicken breast
- 8 ounces of full-Fat: cream cheese, softened
- 1/2 cup of buffalo sauce
- 1/3 cup of full-Fat: ranch dressing
- 1/3 cup of chopped pickled jalapeños
- 1 ½ cups of shredded medium Cheddar cheese, divided
- 2 scallions, sliced

Directions:

1. Put the chicken in a spacious bowl. Remove cream cheese, ranch dressing and buffalo sauce. Stir until they are well blended and mostly smooth with the spices. Fold the jalapeños along with 1 cup of Cheddar.

2. In a 4-cup circular baking dish, add the mixture and add the rest of the Cheddar on top. Place the dish in a basket with a hairdryer.

3. Switch the temperature to 350°F and set the timer for 10 minutes.

4. The top will be brown and bubbling until finished. And cut scallions on top. Serve it hot.

24.Bacon Jalapeño Cheese Bread

Total time: 30 min

Prep time: 10 min

Cook time: 20 min

Yield: 8 sticks (2 sticks per servings)

Ingredients:

- 2 cups of shredded mozzarella cheese
- ¼ cup of grated Parmesan cheese
- ¼ cup of chopped pickled jalapeños
- 2 large eggs
- 4 slices of sugar-free bacon, cooked and chopped

Directions:

1. In a wide bowl, combine all ingredients. To suit your Air Fryer basket, trim a piece of parchment.

2. With a bit of sweat, dampen your hands and spread the mixture out into a circle. This will need to be divided into two smaller cheese pieces of bread, depending on the size of your fryer.

3. In the Air Fryer basket, put the parchment and cheese bread.

4. Change the temperature and set the timer to 320°F for 15 minutes.

5. Flip the bread gently while you have 5 minutes left.

6. The top will be golden brown when fully baked. Serve it hot and drink it!

25.Pizza Rolls

Total time: 30 min

Prep time: 10 min

Cook time: 20 min

Yield: 8 sticks (2 sticks per servings)

Ingredients:

- 2 cups of shredded mozzarella cheese
- 1/2 cup of almond flour 2 large eggs
- 72 slices of pepperoni
- 8 (1-ounce) mozzarella string cheese sticks, cut into 3 pieces
- 2 tablespoons of unsalted butter, melted
- 1/4 teaspoon of garlic powder
- ½ teaspoon of dried parsley
- 2 tablespoons of grated Parmesan cheese

Directions:

1. Place the mozzarella and almond flour in a big, microwave-proof dish. 1-minute microwave. Remove the Bowland mix until a ball of dough emerges. If required, microwave for 30 more seconds.

2. Crack the eggs in the bowl and combine until they form a smooth dough ball. With water, wet your hands and knead the dough briefly.

3. Tear off two large pieces of parchment paper and spray non-stick cooking spray on one side of each one.

4. Between the two boards, put the dough ball, with the sprayed sides facing the dough. To stretch the dough out to a thickness of 1/4', use a rolling pin.

5. To slice into 24 rectangles, use a knife. Put 3 pepperoni slices on each rectangle and 1 piece of string cheese.

6. Fold the rectangle in two, covering the filling with pepperoni and cheese. Closed pinch or roll sides. Cut and insert a strip of parchment in the basket to match the Air Fryer basket. Put the parchment on the rolls.

7. Change the temperature and set the timer to 350°F for 10 minutes.

8. Open the fryer after 5 minutes and rotate the rolls of pizza. Restart the fryer and finish frying until the rolls of pizza are golden.

9. Place butter, garlic powder and parsley in a small bowl. Brush the mixture over baked pizza rolls and sprinkle with parmesan. Eat warm. Serve warm.

27.Bacon Cheeseburger Dip

Total time: 30 min

Prep time: 10 min

Cook time: 20 min

Yield: 4 sticks (2 sticks per servings)

Ingredients:

- 8 ounces of full-Fat: cream cheese
- 1/4 cup of full-Fat: mayonnaise
- 1/4 cup of full-Fat: sour cream
- 1/4 cup of chopped onion
- 1 teaspoon of garlic powder

- 1 tablespoon of Worcestershire sauce 1

- 1/4 cups of shredded medium Cheddar cheese, divided

- ½-pound of cooked 80/20 ground beef

- 6 slices of sugar-free bacon, cooked and crumbled

- 2 large pickle spears, chopped.

Directions:

1. In a large microwave-safe bowl, place the cream cheese and microwave for 45 seconds. Stir in mayonnaise, sour cream, onion, powdered garlic, and one cup of Worcestershire Cheddar sauce. Add the bacon and the ground beef. Sprinkle over leftover Cheddar.

2. Place the bowl in 6 "and put it in the basket of the Air Fryer.

3. Set the temperature to 400° F and adjust the timer for 10 minutes.

4. When the top is golden, bubbling sprinkles the pickles over the dish and serves warm.

28.Pork Rind Tortillas

Total time: 30 min

Prep time: 10 min

Cook time: 20 min

Yield: 4 sticks (2 sticks per servings)

Ingredients:

- 1-ounce of pork rinds

- 3/4 cup of shredded mozzarella cheese

- 2 tablespoons of full-Fat: cream cheese

- 1 large egg

Directions:

1. Mount a food processor with pork rinds and pulse until finely soiled.

2. In a big, secure microwave dish, put the mozzarella. Break-in the cream cheese into small pieces and add to the bowl. Microwave for 30 seconds, or before all forms of cheese are melted, and a ball is quickly blended. Apply the ground pork rinds and the egg to the cheese mixture.

3. Continue to stir until a ball shapes the mixture. If it cools too much and the cheese hardens, so microwave for 10 more seconds.

4. Put aside the dough into four little balls. Between two parchment sheets, put each dough ball and roll onto a 1/4 flat mat.

5. Place tortillas in a single layer Air Fryer basket; if necessary, operate in batches.

6. Fix the temperature to 400° F for 5 minutes and set the timer.

7. The tortillas would become crispy and solid when fully baked. Serve and enjoy it immediately!

29.Mozzarella Sticks

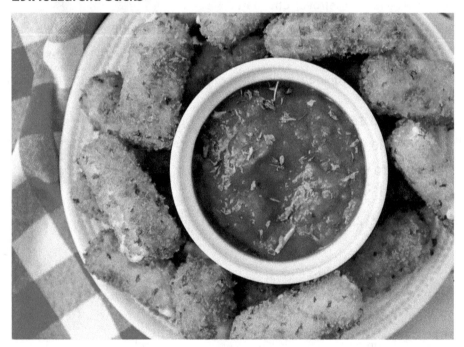

Total time: 30 min

Prep time: 10 min

Cook time: 20 min

Yield: 4 sticks (2 sticks per servings)

Ingredients:

- 6 (1-ounce) mozzarella string cheese sticks
- 1/2 cup of grated Parmesan cheese

- ½- an ounce of pork rinds, finely ground
- 1 teaspoon of dried parsley
- 2 large eggs

Directions:

1. Place the mozzarella sticks on a cutting board and cut them in half. Freeze for 45 minutes or until strong, to stand. When freezing overnight, after 1 hour, cut frozen sticks and place them for future use in an airtight zip-top storage container.

2. In a large bowl, combine the parmesan, ground pork rinds, and parsley together.

3. In a medium cup, whisk the eggs together.

4. Place the frozen mozzarella on top of the beaten eggs, then coat with the Parmesan sauce. For discarded pins, repeat. Place the Air Fryer mozzarella sticks in the bowl.

5. For 10 minutes, change the temperature to 400° F and set the timer to golden.

6. Serve it warm and eat it!

30.Bacon-Wrapped Onion Rings

Total time: 30 min

Prep time: 10 min

Cook time: 20 min

Yield: 4 (2 per servings)

Ingredients:

- 1 large onion, peeled
- 1 tablespoon of sriracha
- 8 slices of sugar-free bacon

Directions:

1. Break the ointment into 1/4-inch thick slices. Take two onion slices and bind the bacon around the loops. For the remaining onion and bacon, repeat.

2. Fix the temperature for 10 minutes to 350° F and adjust the timer.

3. To flip the onion rings halfway through the cooking time, use pliers. Once fully cooked, the bacon will be crispy. Eat hot and enjoy it!

31.Crusted Chicken Tenders

Preparation time: 5 minutes

Cooking time: 15 minutes

Servings: 3

Ingredients:

- ½ cup all-purpose flour
- 2 eggs, beaten
- ½ cup seasoned breadcrumbs
- Salt and freshly ground black pepper, to taste
- 2 tablespoons olive oil
- ¾ pound chicken tenders

Directions:

1. Place the flour in a bowl.
2. Place the eggs in a second bowl.
3. Mix the breadcrumbs, salt, black pepper and oil together in a third dish.
4. Cover the chicken bowls with flour,
5. Dip into the eggs and then coat generously with the combination of breadcrumbs.
6. The air fryer should be preheated to 330 degrees F. Arrange the chicken tenderloin in a basket of air fryers. Cook for 10 minutes, roughly.
7. Set the air fryer to 390 degrees f for now.
8. Cook for 5 more minutes or so.

32.Air Fryer Chicken Parmesan

Preparation time: 5 minutes

Cooking time: 9 minutes

Servings: 4

Ingredients:

- ½ c. Keto marinara
- 6 tbsp. Mozzarella cheese

- 1 tbsp. Melted ghee
- 2 tbsp. Grated parmesan cheese
- 6 tbsp. Gluten-free seasoned breadcrumbs
- 8-ounce chicken breasts

Directions:

1. Make sure you preheat the air fryer to 360 degrees. Using olive oil to mist the basket.

2. Mix the parmesan cheese with the breadcrumbs. Just melt ghee.

3. Brush melted the chicken with ghee and dip into the mixture of breadcrumb.

4. In an air fryer, put the coated chicken and cover it with olive oil.

5. Pour into the rack/basket of the oven. Place the rack on the air fryer's center shelf. Set the temperature to 360 degrees F, and set the time for 6 minutes. Cook 2 breasts for 6 minutes and put a tablespoon of sauce and 11/2 tablespoons of mozzarella cheese on top of each breast. Cook for a further three minutes to melt the cheese.

6. As you replicate the procedure with the remaining breasts, keep the cooked parts warm.

33.Chicken Bbq Recipe from Peru

Preparation time: 5 minutes

Cooking time: 40 minutes

Servings: 4

Ingredients:

- ½ teaspoon dried oregano
- 1 teaspoon paprika
- 1/3 cup soy sauce
- 2 ½ pounds chicken, quartered
- 2 tablespoons fresh lime juice
- 2 teaspoons ground cumin
- 5 cloves of garlic, minced

Directions:

15. After placing all the ingredients in a zip-lock bag, keep the marinade in the refrigerator for 2 hours.

16. Preheat the air fryer to 390°f and place the grilling pan in the air fryer.

17. The chicken has to be grilled for 40 minutes and turn sides every 10 minutes while grilling.

34.Ricotta and Parsley Stuffed Turkey Breasts

Preparation time: 5 minutes

Cooking time: 25 minutes

Servings: 4

Ingredients:

- 1 turkey breast, quartered
- 1 cup ricotta cheese
- 1/4 cup fresh Italian parsley, chopped
- 1 teaspoon garlic powder
- 1/2 teaspoon cumin powder
- 1 egg, beaten
- 1 teaspoon paprika
- Salt and ground black pepper, to taste
- Crushed tortilla chips
- 1 ½ tablespoon extra-virgin olive oil

Directions:

1. Firstly, using a rolling pin, flatten out each slice of turkey breast. Let three mixing bowls packed.

2. Combine the parsley, garlic powder, and cumin powder with the ricotta cheese in a small dish.

3. Place the mixture of ricotta/parsley in the middle of each slice. Repeat and roll them up with the remaining bits of the turkey breast.

4. Whisk the egg along with the paprika in another small dish. Combine the salt, pepper, and smashed tortilla chips in the third small dish.

5. Dip each roll into the whisked egg, then roll it over the mixture of tortilla chips.

6. Move the prepared rolls to the basket of an air fryer. Drizzle the olive oil over everything.

7. Cook for 25 minutes at 350 degrees f, operating in batches. If needed, serve soft, garnished with some extra parsley.

35.Cheesy Turkey-Rice with Broccoli

Preparation time: 5 minutes

Cooking time: 40 minutes

Servings: 4

Ingredients:

- 1 cup cooked, chopped turkey meat
- 1 tablespoon and 1-1/2 teaspoons butter, melted
- 1/2 (10 ounces) package frozen broccoli, thawed
- 1/2 (7 ounces) package whole wheat crackers, crushed
- 1/2 cup shredded cheddar cheese
- 1/2 cup uncooked white rice

Directions:

1. In a saucepan, put 2 cups of water to a boil. Add rice to the mixture and cook for 20 minutes. Turn the fire off and set it aside.
2. Lightly oil the air-fryer baking pan with cooking oil. Combine the fried rice, cheese, ham, and broccoli. To combine, toss well.
3. In a small bowl, combine the melted butter and crushed crackers well. Spread uniformly over the rest of the rice.
4. Pour into the rack/basket of the oven. Place the rack on the air fryer's center shelf. Set the temperature to 360 ° f and set the time to 20 minutes for mild browning of the tops.
5. Serve and enjoy.

36.Jerk Chicken Wings

Preparation time: 10 minutes

Cooking time: 16 minutes

Servings: 6

Ingredients:

- 1 tsp. Salt
- ½ c. Red wine vinegar

- 5 tbsp. Lime juice
- 4 chopped scallions
- 1 tbsp. Grated ginger
- 2 tbsp. Brown sugar
- 1 tbsp. Chopped thyme
- 1 tsp. White pepper
- 1 tsp. Cayenne pepper
- 1 tsp. Cinnamon
- 1 tbsp. Allspice
- 1 habanero pepper (seeds/ribs removed and chopped finely)
- 6 chopped garlic cloves
- 2 tbsp. Low-sodium soy sauce
- 2 tbsp. Olive oil
- 4 pounds of chicken wings

Directions:

1. Combine all the ingredients in a dish, bar the wings. Pour the chicken wings into a gallon bag and add them. To marinate, chill for 2-24 hours.

2. Make sure you preheat your air fryer to 390 degrees F.

3. To remove extra liquids, bring chicken wings into a strainer.

4. Pour half of the wings into the basket of your air fryer. Set the temperature to 390 ° f and set the time to 16 minutes and cook for 14-16 minutes to ensure that you shake halfway through the cooking process.

5. Remove the remaining wings and repeat the process

37. Brazilian Mini Turkey Pies

Preparation Time: 5 Minutes

Cooking Time: 10 Minutes

Servings: 8

Prep + Cook Time: 15 minutes | Servings: 8

Ingredients:

- 1 oz. turkey stock
- 2 oz. whole milk
- 2 oz. coconut milk
- 8 oz. homemade tomato sauce
- 1 tsp. oregano
- 1 tbsp. coriander
- Salt and ground black pepper to taste
- 2 oz. turkey, cooked and shredded
- Flour
- 8 slices filo pastry
- 1 small egg beaten

Directions:

1. Get a clean mixing bowl and put all your wet ingredients, except the egg. Mix well.

2. The result should be a pale-looking sauce – the stock for your pie. Now add the seasoning and turkey before mixing again. Finally, set the mixture aside.

3. To each of your little pie cases, line them with a bit of flour before the filo pastry. This prevents them from sticking. Each pie should use up one sheet of filo, and it should be centrally positioned such that you can easily fold over the extra pastry for the top of the pie.

4. Add the mixture to every mini pie pot until they are ¾ full.

5. Cover the top with the remaining pastry before brushing the egg along the top.

6. Transfer the mini pie pot into the air fryer, set the temperature to 360 F and allow to cook for 10 minutes.

7. Serve

38.Pork Taquitos

Preparation time: 10 minutes

Cooking time: 16 minutes

Servings: 8

Ingredients:

- 1 juiced lime
- 10 whole-wheat tortillas
- 2 ½ c. Shredded mozzarella cheese
- 30 ounces of cooked and shredded pork tenderloin

Directions:

1. Make sure to preheat your air fryer to 380 degrees F.

2. Drizzle pork with lime juice and gently mix.

3. Using a dampened paper towel to smooth the tortillas in the oven.

4. Apply to each tortilla roughly 3 ounces of pork and 1/4 cup of shredded cheese. Wrap them up securely.

5. Spray a little bit of olive oil on the air fryer basket.

6. Set the temperature to 380 degrees F, and set the time for 10 minutes. 7-10 minutes before tortillas turn a faint golden color, make sure to rotate halfway through the cooking process and then enjoy

39.Panko-breaded pork chops

Preparation time: 5 minutes

Cooking time: 12 minutes

Servings: 6

Ingredients:

- 5 (3½- to 5-ounce) pork chops (bone-in or boneless)
- Seasoning salt
- Pepper
- ¼ cup all-purpose flour
- 2 tablespoons panko bread crumbs
- Cooking oil

Directions:

18. Season the pork chops with the seasoning salt and pepper to taste.

19. Sprinkle the flour on both sides of the pork chops, then coat both sides with panko bread crumbs.

20. Place the pork chops in the air fryer. Stacking them is okay.

21. Spray the pork chops with cooking oil. Pour into the oven rack/basket. Place the rack on the middle shelf of the air fryer. Set temperature to 375°f, and set time to 6 minutes. Cook for 6 minutes.

22. Open the air fryer and flip the pork chops. Cook for an additional 6 minutes

23. Cool before serving.

24. Typically, bone-in pork chops are juicier than boneless. If you prefer really juicy pork chops, use bone-in.

40.Apricot glazed pork tenderloins

Preparation time: 5 minutes

Cooking time: 30 minutes

Servings: 3

Ingredients:

- 1 teaspoon salt
- 1/2 teaspoon pepper
- 1-lb pork tenderloin
- 2 tablespoons minced fresh rosemary or 1 tablespoon dried rosemary, crushed
- 2 tablespoons olive oil, divided
- Garlic cloves, minced
- Apricot glaze ingredients:
- 1 cup apricot preserves
- Garlic cloves, minced
- 4 tablespoons lemon juice

Directions:

1. Brush the seasoning or well-mixed seasoning of salt, pepper, garlic and olive oil pork. Pork can be cut into two halves to fit into an air fryer if required.

2. Use cooking spray to grease the air fryer pan and place the port onto it.

3. Cook each side of pork in a preheated 390°f air fryer for 3 minutes.

4. Mix well all of the glaze ingredients in a small bowl.

5. Cook at 330°f for 20 minutes.

6. Serve and enjoy.

41.Barbecue Flavored Pork Ribs

Preparation time: 5 minutes

Cooking time: 15 minutes

Servings: 6

Ingredients:

- ¼ cup honey, divided
- ¾ cup bbq sauce
- 2 tablespoons tomato ketchup
- 1 tablespoon Worcestershire sauce
- 1 tablespoon soy sauce
- ½ teaspoon garlic powder
- Freshly ground white pepper, to taste
- 1¾ pound pork ribs

Directions:

1. In a large bowl, mix together 3 tablespoons of honey and the remaining ingredients except for pork ribs.

2. Refrigerate to marinate for about 20 minutes.

3. Preheat the air fryer to 355 degrees f.

4. Place the ribs in an air fryer basket.

5. Cook for about 13 minutes.

6. Remove the ribs from the air fryer and coat with the remaining honey.

7. Serve hot.

42.Balsamic Glazed Pork Chops

Preparation time: 5 minutes

Cooking time: 50 minutes

Servings: 4

Ingredients:

- ¾ cup balsamic vinegar

- 1 ½ tablespoons sugar
- 1 tablespoon butter
- 3 tablespoons olive oil
- Tablespoons salt
- 3 pork rib chops

Directions:

1. Place all ingredients in a bowl and allow the meat to marinate in the fridge for at least 2 hours.

2. Preheat the air fryer to 390°f.

3. Place the grill pan accessory in the air fryer.

4. Grill the pork chops for 20 minutes, making sure to flip the meat every 10 minutes for even grilling.

5. Meanwhile, pour the balsamic vinegar on a saucepan and allow to simmer for at least 10 minutes until the sauce thickens.

6. Brush the meat with the glaze before serving.

43.Rustic Pork Ribs

Preparation time: 5 minutes

Cooking time: 15 minutes

Servings: 4

Ingredients:

- 1 rack of pork ribs
- 3 tablespoons dry red wine
- 1 tablespoon soy sauce
- 1/2 teaspoon dried thyme
- 1/2 teaspoon onion powder
- 1/2 teaspoon garlic powder
- 1/2 teaspoon ground black pepper
- 1 teaspoon smoked salt
- 1 tablespoon cornstarch
- 1/2 teaspoon olive oil

Directions:

1. First, preheat your air fryer to 390 degrees f. Marinate after mixing all the ingredients for at least 1 hour.

2. Set temperature to 390°f, for 25 minutes and place the rack on the middle shelf of the air fryer. Cook the ribs for almost 25 minutes.

3. Serve hot.

44.Keto Parmesan Crusted Pork Chops

Preparation time: 10 minutes

Cooking time: 15 minutes

Servings: 8

Ingredients:

- 3 tbsp. Grated parmesan cheese
- 1 c. Pork rind crumbs
- 2 beaten eggs
- ¼ tsp. Chili powder
- ½ tsp. Onion powder
- 1 tsp. Smoked paprika
- ¼ tsp. Pepper
- ½ tsp. Salt
- 4-6 thick boneless pork chops

Directions:

1. Preheat your air fryer to 400 degrees F.

2. Season all sides of the pork chops with pepper and salt.

3. Pulse pork rinds into crumbs in a food processor. And other seasonings, combine the crumbs.

4. Whip the eggs and add them to another bowl.

5. Dip pork chops into eggs and then into a combination of pork rind crumbs.

6. Spray the olive oil on an air fryer and add the pork chops to the basket. Set the temperature to 400 degrees F, and set the time for 15 minutes.

45.Crispy Fried Pork Chops the Southern Way

Preparation time: 10 minutes

Cooking time: 25 minutes

Servings: 4

Ingredients:

- ½ cup all-purpose flour
- ½ cup low-fat buttermilk
- ½ teaspoon black pepper
- ½ teaspoon tabasco sauce
- Teaspoon paprika
- 3 bone-in pork chops

Directions:

1. In a zip-lock bag, put the buttermilk and the hot sauce and add the pork chops. Enable it to marinate in the fridge for at least an hour.
2. Combine the rice, paprika, and black pepper in a dish.
3. Let the pork out of the zip-lock container and dredge it with the flour mixture.
4. Preheat to 390°f with the air fryer.
5. With cooking oil, brush the pork chops.
6. Pour into the rack/basket of the oven. Place the rack on the air fryer's center shelf. Set the temperature to 390 degrees F, and set the time for 25 minutes.

46.Scrumptious Rib-Eye Steak

Preparation time: 5 minutes

Cooking time: 15 minutes

Servings: 2

Ingredients:

- 2 rib-eye steaks, sliced 1 1/2- inch pieces
- 1/2 cup soy sauce
- 1/4 cup olive oil
- 4 teaspoons grill seasoning

Directions:

1. Combine the steaks, salt, olive oil and soy sauce in a resealable bag; shake to cover well and allow to marinate for at least 2 hours.

2. Pick the meat and discard the marinade from the bag.

3. The air fryer toast oven pan is added with a splash of water and then preheated to 400 degrees.

4. In the basket, add the meat and simmer for 7 minutes. Switch the steak over and cook for an extra 8 minutes. Remove the meat and leave to rest before serving for at least 5 minutes.

47.Air Fryer Toast Oven Sticky Pork Ribs

Preparation time: 2-12 hours

Cooking time: 15 minutes

Servings: 4

Ingredients:

- 1 rack pork baby back ribs
- 1 tbsp. Oyster sauce
- 2 tbsp. Light soy sauce
- 1 tsp. Dark soy sauce
- 1 tbsp. Mustard
- 1 ½ tbsp. Pure honey
- 5 cloves garlic, halved
- 1-inch fresh garlic, sliced
- For the sauce:
- 1 tbsp. Soy sauce
- 1 tbsp. Fish sauce
- 2 tsp. Toasted rice powder
- 1 tsp. Sugar
- 2 tsp. Red chili flakes
- Freshly squeezed juice of ½ a lemon
- 2 tsp. Finely chopped cilantro
- 1 clove garlic, finely chopped

Directions:

1. To make the marinade, mix all the ingredients for the ribs in a dish, apart from the ribs.

2. Separate the ribs and put the marinade in a wide bowl over the ribs, ensuring that the ribs are well protected. Cover with adhesive tape and marinate for at least 2 hours. Marinate overnight for better results.

3. Set 360 degrees f for your air fryer toast oven,

4. In the air-fryer toast oven, add the ribs, garlic and ginger bits. Do not stir in the juices. Six minutes to prepare, shake well and 6 more minutes to cook.

5. Create the dip by adding all the sauce ingredients while the ribs cook: then set it aside in a small dish.

6. With the dipping sauce, relish the ribs.

7. Enjoy!

48.Coriander Lamb with Pesto' N Mint Dip

Preparation time: 5 minutes

Cooking time: 15 minutes

Servings: 4

Ingredients:

- 1 1/2 teaspoons coriander seeds, ground in a spice mill or mortar with a pestle

- 1 large red bell pepper, cut into 1-inch squares

- 1 small red onion, cut into 1-inch squares

- 1 tablespoon extra-virgin olive oil plus additional for brushing

- 1 teaspoon coarse kosher salt

- 1-pound trimmed lamb meat, cut into 1 1/4-inch cube

- 4 large garlic cloves, minced

- Mint-pesto dip ingredients:

- 1 cup (packed) fresh mint leaves

- 2 tablespoons pine nuts

- 2 tablespoons freshly grated parmesan cheese

- 1 tablespoon fresh lemon juice

- 1 medium garlic clove, peeled

- 1/2 cup (packed) fresh cilantro leaves

- 1/2 teaspoon coarse kosher salt

- 1/2 cup (or more) extra-virgin olive oil

Directions:

1. Puree all the dip ingredients in the blender until smooth and fluffy. Transfer and set aside in a bowl.

2. Mix the coriander, salt, garlic, and oil in a wide cup. Add lamb, toss to cover well. Marinate in the ref for a minimum of an hour.

3. In a skewer, thread the lamb, bell pepper, and onion alternately. Repeat until all ingredients are complete: re-use. Place it in the air fryer on the skewer rack.

4. Cook on 390 halfway through cooking time, turnover, for 8 minutes,

5. Serve on the side and eat with sauce.

49.Cumin-Sichuan Lamb Bbq with Dip

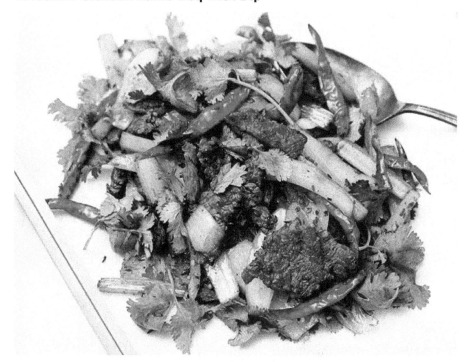

Preparation time: 10 minutes

Cooking time: 25 minutes

Servings: 4

Ingredients:

- 1 1/4 pounds boneless lamb shoulder, cut into 1-inch pieces
- 1 tablespoon Sichuan peppercorns or 1 teaspoon black peppercorns
- 1 teaspoon sugar
- 2 tablespoons cumin seeds
- 2 teaspoons caraway seeds
- 2 teaspoons crushed red pepper flakes
- Finely grated lemon zest (for serving)
- Kosher salt, freshly cracked pepper
- For the garlic yogurt dip:
- 1 garlic clove, grated
- 1 tablespoon fresh lemon juice
- 1 cup plain greek yogurt
- Kosher salt, freshly ground pepper
- 1/2 teaspoon finely grated lemon zest

Directions:

1. Process the cumin seeds, peppercorns, caraway seeds, pepper flakes and sugar in a food processor until smooth.
2. Thread bits of lamb into skewers. With salt, season. Rub the paste all over the bits of meat.
3. Place the rack on the skewer.
4. Cook at 390 or to the optimal density for 5 minutes.
5. Meanwhile, whisk the ingredients well in a medium bowl and set aside.
6. Serve with dip and enjoy.

50.Garlic Lemon-Wine on Lamb Steak

Preparation time: 20 minutes

Cooking time: 1 hour and 30 minutes

Servings: 4

Ingredients:

- ¼ cup extra virgin olive oil
- ½ cup dry white wine
- 1 tablespoon brown sugar
- 2 pounds lamb steak, pounded
- 2 tablespoons lemon juice
- 3 tablespoons ancho chili powder
- 8 cloves of garlic, minced
- Salt and pepper to taste

Directions:

1. Place all the ingredients in a bowl and let the meat marinate for at least 2 hours in the refrigerator.
2. To 390f, preheat the air fryer.
3. Place the accessory for the grill pan in the air-fryer.
4. For 20 minutes per batch, grill the beef.
5. Meanwhile, in a saucepan, pour the marinade and let it boil for 10 minutes before the sauce thickens.

51.Garlic-Rosemary Lamb Bbq

Preparation time: 5 minutes

Cooking time: 12 minutes

Servings: 2

Ingredients:

- 1-lb cubed lamb leg
- Juice of 1 lemon
- Fresh rosemary
- 3 smashed garlic cloves
- Salt and pepper
- 1/2 cup olive oil

Directions:

1. Mix all the ingredients in a shallow bowl, and marinate for 3 hours.

2. Thread bits of lamb into skewers. Place it in an air fryer on a skewer rack.

3. Cook at 390F for 12 minutes. Turnover skewers, halfway through cooking time. Cook in batches if needed.

4. Enjoy and serve.

52. Maras Pepper Lamb Kebab Recipe from Turkey

Preparation time: 5 minutes

Cooking time: 15 minutes

Servings: 2

Ingredients:

- 1-lb lamb meat, cut into 2-inch cubes

- Kosher salt

- Freshly cracked black pepper

- 2 tablespoons maras pepper, or 2 teaspoons other dried chili powder mixed with 1 tablespoon paprika

- 1 teaspoon minced garlic

- 2 tablespoons roughly chopped fresh mint

- 1/2 cup extra-virgin olive oil, divided

- 1/2 cup dried apricots, cut into medium dice

Directions:

1. Combine the pepper, salt, and half of the olive oil in a cup. To coat, add lamb and toss well. Thread out 4 skewers of lamb.

2. Cook at 390 or to the optimal density for 5 minutes.

3. Mix well the remaining oil, mint, garlic, maras pepper, and apricots in a wide bowl. Add the lamb roasted. With salt and pepper, season. Toss well, coat,

4. Enjoy and serve.

53. Saffron Spiced Rack of Lamb

Preparation time: 20 minutes

Cooking time: 1 hour and 10 minutes

Servings: 4

Ingredients:

- ½ teaspoon crumbled saffron threads
- 1 cup plain greek yogurt
- 1 teaspoon lemon zest
- 2 cloves of garlic, minced
- 2 racks of lamb, rib bones frenched
- 2 tablespoons olive oil
- Salt and pepper to taste

Directions:

1. To 390f, preheat the air fryer.
2. Place the accessory for the grill pan in the air-fryer.
3. With salt and pepper to taste, season the lamb meat. Only set aside.
4. Combine the remaining ingredients in a dish.
5. Brush the mixture onto the lamb.
6. Set aside and cook for 1 hour and 10 minutes on the grill pan.

54.Shepherd's Pie Made Of Ground Lamb

Preparation time: 20 minutes

Cooking time: 50 minutes

Servings: 4

Ingredients:

- 1-pound lean ground lamb
- 2 tablespoons and 2 teaspoons all-purpose flour
- Salt and ground black pepper to taste
- 1 teaspoon minced fresh rosemary
- 2 tablespoons cream cheese
- 2 ounces Irish cheese (such as dubliner®), shredded
- Salt and ground black pepper to taste

- 1 tablespoon milk
- 1-1/2 teaspoons olive oil
- 1-1/2 teaspoons butter
- 1/2 onion, diced
- 1/2 teaspoon paprika
- 1-1/2 teaspoons ketchup
- 1-1/2 cloves garlic, minced
- 1/2 (12 ounces) package frozen peas and carrots, thawed
- 1-1/2 teaspoons butter
- 1/2 pinch ground cayenne pepper
- 1/2 egg yolk
- 1-1/4 cups water, or as needed
- 1-1/4 pounds Yukon gold potatoes, peeled and halved
- 1/8 teaspoon ground cinnamon

Directions:

1. Boil a big saucepan of salted water and add the potatoes. Simmer until tender, for 15 minutes.

2. Meanwhile, gently grease the air-fryer baking pan with butter. Melt at 360f for 2 minutes.

3. Mix ground lamb and onion. Cook for 10 minutes, halfway through cooking time, stirring and crumbling.

4. Garlic, ketchup, cinnamon, paprika, black pepper, rosemary, salt, and flour are added. Mix thoroughly and cook for 3 minutes.

5. Add water and pan deglaze. For 6 minutes, continue cooking.

6. Stir in the peas and carrots. Spread the mixture uniformly in the pan.

7. Drain well once the potatoes are finished and move the potatoes to a bowl. Mash the potatoes and stir in the cream cheese, cayenne pepper, butter and Irish cheese. Mix thoroughly. To taste, season with pepper and salt.

8. Whisk the milk and egg yolk well in a small cup. Stir the mashed potatoes in.

9. Top the mixture of ground lamb with mashed potatoes.

10. Cook for an additional 15 minutes or until the potato tops are lightly browned.

11. Enjoy and serve.

55.Simple Lamb Bbq with Herbed Salt

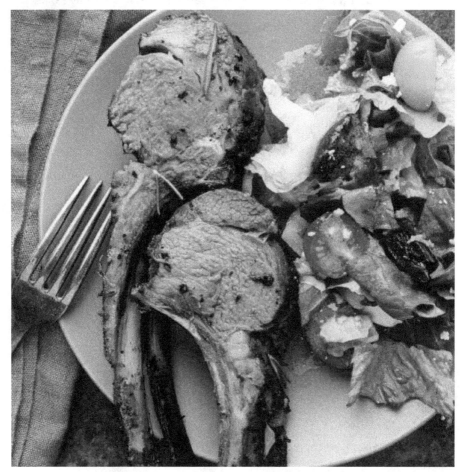

Preparation time: 20 minutes

Cooking time: 1 hour 20 minutes

Servings: 8

Ingredients:

- 2 ½ tablespoons herb salt
- 2 tablespoons olive oil

- 4 pounds boneless leg of lamb, cut into 2-inch chunks

Directions:

1. Preheat the air fryer to 390 f.

2. Place the grill pan accessory in the air fryer.

3. Season the meat with the herb salt and brush with olive oil.

4. Grill the meat for 20 minutes per batch.

5. Make sure to flip the meat every 10 minutes for even cooking.

56.Greek Lamb Meatballs

Preparation time: 12 minutes

Cooking time: 12 minutes

Servings: 12

Ingredients:

- 1 pound ground lamb
- ½ cup breadcrumbs
- ¼ cup milk
- 2 egg yolks
- 1 teaspoon ground coriander
- 1 teaspoon ground cumin
- 3 garlic cloves, minced
- 1 teaspoon dried oregano
- ½ teaspoon salt
- ½ teaspoon black pepper
- 1 lemon, juiced and zested
- ¼ cup fresh parsley, chopped
- ½ cup crumbled feta cheese
- Olive oil, for shaping
- Tzatziki, for dipping

Directions:

1. Combine all ingredients except olive oil in a large mixing bowl and mix well.

2. Form 12 meatballs, about 2 ounces each. Use olive oil on your hands, so they don't stick to the meatballs. Set aside.

3. Select the broil function on the cosori air fryer toaster oven, set the time to 12 minutes, then press the start/cancel to preheat.

4. Place the meatballs on the food tray, then insert the tray at the top position in the preheated air fryer toaster oven. Press start/cancel.

5. Take out the meatballs when done and serve with a side of tzatziki.

57.Lamb Gyro

Preparation time: 10 minutes

Cooking time: 25 minutes

Servings: 4

Ingredients:

- 1 pound ground lamb
- Tzatziki sauce, to taste
- ¼ red onion, minced
- ¼ cup mint, minced
- ½ teaspoon black pepper
- 12 mint leaves, minced
- 4 slices of pita bread
- ¾ cup hummus
- 1 cup romaine lettuce, shredded
- ½ onion sliced
- 2 cloves garlic, minced
- ½ teaspoon salt
- 1 Roma tomato, diced
- ½ cucumber, skinned and thinly sliced
- ¼ cup parsley, minced
- ⅛ teaspoon rosemary

Directions:

1. Mix ground lamb, red onion, mint, parsley, garlic, salt, rosemary, and black pepper until fully combined.

2. Select the broil function on the cosori air fryer toaster oven, set time to 25 minutes and temperature to 450°f, then press the start/cancel to preheat.

3. Line the food tray with parchment paper and place the ground lamb on top, shaping it into a patty 1-inch-thick and 6 inches in diameter.

4. Insert the food tray at the top position in the preheated air fryer toaster oven, then press the start/cancel.

5. Remove when done and cut into thin slices.

6. Assemble each gyro starting with pita bread, then hummus, lamb meat, lettuce, onion, tomato, cucumber, and mint leaves, drizzle with tzatziki.

7. Serve immediately.

58.Masala Galette

Total time: 30 min

Prep time: 10 min

Cook time: 25 min

Yield: 2 servings

Ingredients:

- 2 tbsp. of garam masala
- 2 medium potatoes boiled and mashed
- 1 ½ cup of coarsely crushed peanuts
- 3 tsp. of ginger finely chopped
- 1-2 tbsp. of fresh coriander leaves
- 2 or 3 green chilies finely chopped
- 1 ½ tbsp. of lemon juice
- Salt and pepper to taste

Directions:

1. Blend into a clean container with the ingredients.

2. Shape this mixture into galettes that are smooth and round.

3. Wet the galettes softly with sweat. Fill each galette with crushed peanuts.

4. Preheat the Air Fryer, at 160° Fahrenheit, for 5 minutes. Place your basket galettes and let them steam at the bottom for another 25 minutes.

5. At the same temperature, just. Go turn them over to cook them. Using ketchup or mint chutney to serve.

59.Potato Samosa

Total time:30 min

Prep time: 10 min

Cook time:20 min

Yield:6 servings

Ingredients:

For wrappers:

- 2 tbsp. of unsalted butter
- 1 ½ cup of all-purpose flour
- A pinch of salt to taste
- Add as much water as required to make the dough stiff and firm

For filling:

- 2-3 big potatoes boiled and mashed
- ¼ cup of boiled peas
- 1 tsp. of powdered ginger
- 1 or 2 green chilies that are finely chopped or mashed
- ½ tsp. of cumin
- 1 tsp. of coarsely crushed coriander
- 1 dry red chili broken into pieces
- A small amount of salt (to the taste)
- ½ tsp. of dried mango powder
- ½ tsp. of red chili powder.
- 1-2 tbsp. Of coriander.

Directions:

1. To keep it stiff to smooth for external wrapping, rub the dough. When the filling is finished, let it rest in a pot.

2. In a saucepan, heat the ingredients and combine well to make a sticky paste. Write the bread out.

3. Cover and flatten the dough into cubes. Break them in half and add the filling afterward. To support you, fold the rims to make a cone shape, use water.

4. For around 5-6 minutes, preheat the Air Fryer at 300 Fahrenheit. Put all the samosas in the basket and shut the basket properly. Hold the Air Fryer, at 200°, for another 20 to 25 minutes.

5. At the halfway point, open the basket, and turn the samosas over for regular preparation. Fry at 250 ° for around 10 minutes after this, to give them the ideal golden-brown shade. Wet to serve. Recommended sides have tamarind or mint chutney.

6.

60.Vegetable Kebab

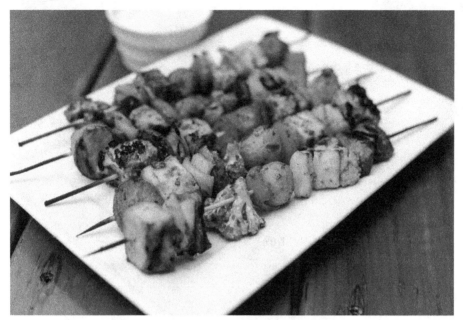

Total time: 30 min

Prep time: 10 min

Cook time: 20 min

Yield: 2 servings

Ingredients:

- 2 cups of mixed vegetables
- 3 onions chopped
- 5 green chilies-roughly chopped
- 1 ½ tbsp. of ginger paste
- 1 ½ tsp. of garlic paste
- 1 ½ tsp. of salt
- 3 tsp. of lemon juice
- 2 tsp. of garam masala
- 4 tbsp. of chopped coriander
- 3 tbsp. of cream

- 3 tbsp. of chopped capsicum
- 3 eggs
- 2 ½ tbsp. of white sesame seeds

Directions:

1. Grind the ingredients, except for the egg, and make a smooth paste. Coat the paste goods with the mask. Now, pound the eggs and add more salt to them.

2. Scatter the coated vegetables in the egg mixture, then transfer to the sesame seeds and garnish well with herbs. Place them on a stick with the vegetables.

3. Pre-fire the Air Fryer at 160 ° Fahrenheit for roughly 5 minutes. Place the sticks in the basket and simmer for 25 more minutes.

4. Move the clamps to the cook's suite during the cooking process, only at the same temperature.

61.Sago Galette

Total time: 25 min

Prep time: 10 min

Cook time: 25 min

Yield: 2 servings

Ingredients:

- 2 cups of sago soaked
- 1 ½ cup of coarsely crushed peanuts
- 3 tsp. of ginger finely chopped
- 1-2 tbsp. of fresh coriander leaves
- 2 or 3 green chilies finely chopped
- 1 ½ tbsp. of lemon juice
- Salt and pepper to the taste

Directions:

1. Wash the soaked sago with the other ingredients, and place it in a clean tub. Shape this mixture into flat and round galettes.

2. Wet the galettes softly with sweat. Fill each galette with crushed peanuts.

3. Preheat the Air Fryer, at 160° Fahrenheit, for 5 minutes. Place your fry basket galettes and allow them to steam at the bottom, just the same temperature for another 25 minutes. Go to fry and turn them over. Serve with chutney, basil or ketchup.

62.Stuffed Capsicum Baskets

Total time: 25 min

Prep time: 10 min

Cook time: 25 min

Yield: 2 servings

Ingredients:

For baskets:

- 3-4 long capsicum
- ½ tsp. ot salt
- ½ tsp. of pepper powder

For filling:

- 1 medium onion finely chopped
- 1 green chili finely chopped
- 2 or 3 large potatoes boiled and mashed
- 1 ½ tbsp. of chopped coriander leaves
- 1 tsp. of fenugreek
- 1 tsp. of dried mango powder
- 1 tsp. of cumin powder
- Salt and pepper to the taste

For topping:

- 3 tbsp. of grated cheese
- 1 tsp. of red chili flakes
- ½ tsp. of oregano
- ½ tsp. of basil
- ½ tsp. of parsley

Directions:

1. Take all the ingredients under the heading "Filling." and put them together in a pan.

2. Cut off the stem of the capsicum. Break out the caps. Remove the seeds as well.

3. Sprinkle over the capsicum inside with some salt and pepper. Switch on, until some time ago, and they were apart.

4. Now fill the intended filling with the hollowed-out capsicums. Sprinkle with the grated cheese, and still add the seasoning.

5. Preheat at 140 ° Fahrenheit for 5 minutes with the Air Fryer. Place the capsicums in and around the basket of fried rice. Let them cook 20 more minutes more temperature, as well. Turn them to hide from cooking in between.

63.Baked Macaroni Pasta

Total time: 25 min

Prep time: 10 min

Cook time: 25 min

Yield: 2 servings

Ingredients:

- 1 cup of pasta
- 7 cups of boiling water
- 1 ½ tbsp. of olive oil
- A pinch of salt

For tossing pasta:

- 1 ½ tbsp. of olive oil
- ½ cup of small carrot pieces
- Salt and pepper to the taste
- ½ tsp. of oregano
- ½ tsp. of basil

For the white sauce:

- 2 tbsp. of olive oil
- 2 tbsp. of all-purpose flour
- 2 cups of milk

- 1 tsp. of dried oregano

- ½ tsp. of dried basil

- ½ tsp. of dried parsley

- Salt and pepper to the taste

Directions:

- Cook the pasta and sieve when finished. Toss the pasta with the ingredients mentioned above and set aside. For the sauce, add the ingredients to a skillet and bring them to a boil.

- To produce a thicker sauce, drop the sauce and begin to boil. Connect the pasta to the sauce and put it in a glass dish garnished with cheese.

- Preheat the Air Fryer, at 160°, for 5 minutes. Place the basket in the bowl and fasten it. Let it proceed to boil for 10 minutes at the same temperature. Hold the sauce, stirring.

64.Macaroni Samosa

Total time: 30 min

Prep time: 10 min

Cook time: 10 min

Yield: 2 servings

Ingredients:

For wrappers:

- 1 cup of all-purpose flour

- 2 tbsp. of unsalted butter

- A pinch of salt to the taste

- Take the amount of water sufficient enough to make a stiff dough

For filling:

- 3 cups of boiled macaroni

- 2 onion sliced

- 2 capsicum sliced

- 2 carrot sliced

- 2 cabbage sliced

- 2 tbsp. of soya sauce

- 2 tsp. of vinegar

- 2 tbsp. of ginger finely chopped

- 2 tbsp. of garlic finely chopped

- 2 tbsp. of green chilies finely chopped

- 2 tbsp. of ginger-garlic paste

- Some salt and pepper to taste

- 2 tbsp. of olive oil

- ½ tsp. of Ajinomoto

Directions:

1. To keep it stiff to smooth for external wrapping, rub the dough. When the filling is full, set the remainder aside in a bowl.

2. In a saucepan, heat the ingredients and combine well to make a sticky paste. Let the color work out.

3. Cover and flatten the dough into cubes. Halve the break-in, then add the filling. To support you, fold the rims to make a cone shape, use water.

4. For around 5-6 minutes, preheat the Air Fryer at 300 Fahrenheit. Place all the samosas in one place, then lock the basket properly. Hold the Air Fryer, at 200°, for another 20 to 25 minutes.

5. Open the bowl and turn over the samosas to cook them uniformly. Afterward, fry at 250 ° for about 10 minutes to give them the perfect golden tan shade. Wet to serve. Tamarinds or green chutney includes the recommended sides.

65.Burritos

Total time: 35 min

Prep time: 10 min

Cook time: 15 min

Yield: 2 servings

Ingredients:

Refried beans:

- ½ cup of red kidney beans (soaked overnight)

- ½ small onion chopped
- 1 tbsp. of olive oil
- 2 tbsp. of tomato puree
- ¼ tsp. of red chili powder
- 1 tsp. of salt to the taste
- 4-5 flour tortillas

Vegetable Filling:

- 1 tbsp. of olive oil
- 1 medium onion finely sliced
- 3 flakes of garlic crushed
- ½ cup of French beans (Slice them lengthwise into thin and long slices)
- ½ cup of mushrooms thinly sliced
- 1 cup of cottage cheese cut in too long and slightly thick fingers
- ½ cup of shredded cabbage
- 1 tbsp. of coriander, chopped
- 1 tbsp. of vinegar
- 1 tsp. of white wine
- A pinch of salt to the taste
- ½ tsp. of red chili flakes
- 1 tsp. of freshly ground peppercorns
- ½ cup of pickled jalapenos (Chop them up finely)
- 2 carrots (Cut into long thin slices)

Salad:

- 1-2 lettuce leaves shredded.
- 1 or 2 spring onions chopped finely. Also, cut the greens.
- 1 tomato. Remove the seeds and chop them into small pieces.
- 1 green chili chopped.
- 1 cup of cheddar cheese, grated.

Directions:

1. Cook the beans along with the onion and garlic and mash them finely. Now, prepare the burrito sauce you're going to need. Make sure you make a sauce that is slightly thick.

2. You may need to cook the ingredients well in a pan for the filling and to ensure that the vegetables on the outside are browned.

3. Place the tortilla and apply a layer of salsa, followed by the beans and the filling in the middle. To make the salad, toss the ingredients together. You'll need to put the salad on top of the filling before rolling it out.

4. At 200 Fahrenheit, preheat the Air Fryer for about 5 minutes. Keep the burritos inside and open the fry basket. Cover the basket accordingly. For another 15 minutes or so, let the Air Fryer sit at 200 Fahrenheit.

5. Remove the basket and turn all the burritos over halfway through, and get a uniform chef.

66.Cheese and Bean Enchiladas

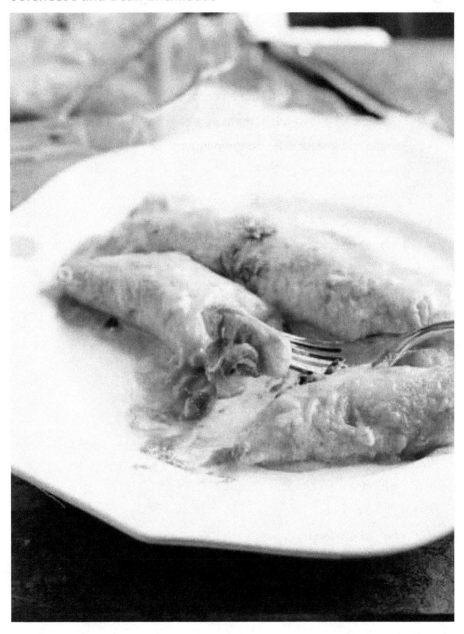

Total time: 35 min

Prep time: 10 min

Cook time: 15 min

Yield: 2 servings

Ingredients:

- Flour tortillas (as many as required)

Red sauce:

- 4 tbsp. of olive oil
- 1 ½ tsp. of garlic that has been chopped
- 1 ½ cups of readymade tomato puree
- 3 medium tomatoes. Puree them in a mixer
- 1 tsp. of sugar
- A pinch of salt or to the taste
- A few red chili flakes to sprinkle
- 1 tsp. of oregano

Filling:

- 2 tbsp. of oil
- 2 tsp. of chopped garlic
- 2 onions chopped finely
- 2 capsicums chopped finely
- 2 cups of readymade baked beans
- A few drops of Tabasco sauce
- 1 cup of crumbled or roughly mashed cottage cheese (cottage cheese)
- 1 cup of grated cheddar cheese
- A pinch of salt
- 1 tsp. of oregano
- ½ tsp. of pepper
- 1 ½ tsp. of red chili flakes or to taste
- 1 tbsp. of finely chopped jalapenos

To serve:

- 1 cup of grated pizza cheese (mix mozzarella and cheddar cheese)

Directions:

1. Have the tortillas ready to serve.

2. Now, move on to the making of red sauce. Put about 2 teaspoons in a saucepan: apply the garlic to heat and whisk. Under the heading "For the sauce," Keep working, apply the remaining ingredients. Cook until the drops of sauce become dense.

3. To fill another saucepan, heat one tablespoon of oil. Tie the onions and garlic together, then fry until caramelized or golden-brown. Put the remainder of the ingredients into the filling and cook for two minutes.

4. From the flame, take the saucepan and grate some cheese over the pan. Balance well, and allow a little bit of it to settle.

5. Let's get a selection of platters. Take a tortilla, then apply some sauce to the surface. Now place the filling at the right, in a line. Turn the tortilla upwards cautiously. And the same is those around tortillas.

6. Place all the tortillas in a bowl and sprinkle them with the grated cheese. Cover all up with an aluminum board.

7. Preheat at 160 ° C for 4-5 minutes with the Air Fryer. Smash the bowl and the tray inside. At the same time, keep the fryer on for another 15 minutes. Switch the tortillas over in between to get a regular chef.

67.Veg Memo's

Total time: 30 min

Prep time: 10 min

Cook time: 10 min

Yield: 2 servings

Ingredients:

For dough:

- 1 ½ cup of all-purpose flour
- ½ tsp. of salt or to taste
- 5 tbsp. of water

For filling:

- 2 cups of carrots grated
- 2 cups of cabbage grated

- 2 tbsp. of oil

- 2 tsp. of ginger-garlic paste

- 2 tsp. of soy sauce

- 2 tsp. of vinegar

Directions:

1. Setback, knead and cover the dough with plastic wrap. Then, cook the filling ingredients and aim to ensure that the sauce is properly coated with the vegetables.

2. Print the dough out and then slice it into a rectangle. Place the filling in the middle. To safeguard the filling, fold the dough now, then pinch the corners.

3. Preheat at 200 ° F for 5 minutes with the Air Fryer. Place the gnocchi in the frying box and close it. Let them cook at the same time for another 20 minutes. The suggested sides contain chili or sauce with ketchup.

68.Yummy Pollock

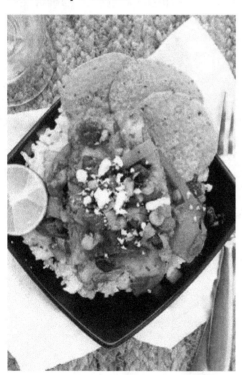

Total time: 25 min

Prep time: 15 min

Cook time: 10 min

Yield: 6 serving

Ingredients:

- Cup 1/2 sour cream
- Four Pollock fillets, barefoot
- Parmesan: 1/4 cup, rubbed
- 2 Mezzanine sugar, melted
- Salt and black chili, to try
- Kitchen spray

Directions:

1. Mix the sour cream in a dish of butter, parmesan, salt and pepper and Whisk well.

2. Sprinkle fish with spray to fry, and season with salt and pepper.

3. Place sour cream mixture on each side. Arrange Pollock fillet in air fryer heated to 350 degrees F, then cook for 15 minutes.

4. Divide Pollock fillets into bowls, and serve with a delightful side salad.

69.Honey Sea Bass

Total time: 40 min

Prep time: 15 min

Cook time: 25 min

Yield: 2 serving

Ingredients:

- 2 Fillets sea bass
- A 1/2 orange zest, rubbed
- 1/2 Fruit juice
- A tablespoon of black pepper and salt
- 2 Mustard spoons
- 2 Honey Teaspoons

- 2 Pounds of olive oil
- 1/2 pound of dried, drained lentils
- A tiny amount of dill, chopped
- 2 Ounces of cress water
- A tiny amount of chopped parsley

Directions:

1. Add salt and peppered fish fillets, apply citrus zest and juice, and rub

Rub with 1 spoonful of milk, honey and mustard, and pass to your air

Fry and cook for 10 minutes at 350 degrees F, turning in half.

2. In the meantime, place the lentils in a small pot, heat them up over medium heat, and add them

Staying with milk, watercress, dill and parsley, mix well and split between

Plates.

3. Insert the fish fillets and serve promptly.

Enjoy it!

Nutrition: 212 calories, 8 fat, 12 fiber, 9 carbohydrates and 17 proteins

70.Tilapia Sauce and Chives
Total time: 20 min

Prep time: 10 min

Cook time: 10 min

Yield: 4 serving

Ingredients:

- 4 Medium fillet with tilapia
- Cooking spray
- Salt and black chili, to satisfy
- 2 Honey Teaspoons
- Greek yoghurt: 1/4 cup
- 1 lemon juice
- 2 Spoonful's of chives, chopped

Directions:

1. Season with salt and pepper, sprinkle with mist, put in

Hot oven 350 degrees F air fryer and cook for ten minutes, tossing

Midway.

2. In the meantime, blend yoghurt with sugar, salt, vinegar, vinegar and chives in a cup

Nice lemon juice and whisk.

3. Divide air fryer fish into bowls, chop yoghurt sauce and serve

Immediately.

Experience!

Nutrition: 261 calories, fat 8, 18 fiber, 24 carbohydrates, 21 protein

71.Tilapia Coconut

Prep time: ten minutes Cooking time: 10 minutes Servings: 4

Ingredients:

- 4 Medium fillet with tilapia
- Salt and black chili, to try
- 1/2 cup of cocoon milk
- 1 Ginger-spoon, rubbed
- Chopped 1/2 cup cilantro
- 2 Sliced cloves of garlic
- 1/2 teaspoon masala garam
- Cooking spray
- Half Jalapeno, Split

Directions:

1. Mix the coconut milk with salt, pepper, cilantro in your food processor,

Ginger, garlic, jalapeno which masala garam, and always pulse well.

2. Sprinkle fish with cooking oil, scatter coconut mix around, rub well,

Switch to the basket with the air fryer and cook at 400 degrees F for 10

Minutes.

3. Divide between plates, and serve hot.

Experience!

Nutrition: 200 calories, 5 fat, 6 fiber, 25 carbohydrates and 26 protein

72.Catfish fillets special
Total time: 40 min

Prep time: 15 min

Cook time: 25 min

Yield: 5 serving

Ingredients:

- 2 Catfish fillets
- 1/2 Teaspoon of ginger, hazelnut
- 2 Butter on ounces
- Worcestershire 4 ounces sauce
- 1/2 cubicle jerk seasoning
- 1 Mustard casserole
- 1 spoonful of balsamic vinegar
- Catsup: 3/4 cup
- Salt and black chili, to try
- 1 spoonful of parsley, chopped

Directions:

1. Heat up a skillet over medium heat with the butter, add Worcestershire

Seasoning of sauce, garlic, mustard, catsup, vinegar, salt and hot pepper,

Adjust fire, swirl well, and apply fish fillets.

2. Toss well, leave the fillets for 10 minutes, drain them, and pass them to the preheated to 350 degrees F air fryer basket and cook for 8 minutes,

Halfway through flip fillets.

3. Divide into bowls, brush on top with parsley and serve immediately.

73.Tasty French Cod
Total time: 30 min

Prep time: 15 min

Cook time: 15 min

Yield: 6 serving

Ingredients:

- 2 Tsp. of olive oil
- 1 Yellow onion, Sliced
- White wine: 1/2 cup
- 2 cloves of garlic, minced
- 14 Ounces of dried, stewed tomatoes
- Chopped 3 teaspoons of parsley
- 2 Lbs. of cod, boneless
- Salt and black chili, to try
- 2 tablespoons of butter

Directions:

1. Heat a saucepan over medium heat with the oil, add garlic and onion, stir and just cook for five minutes.

2. Add wine, stir and proceed to cook for 1 minute.

3. Stir in tomatoes, bring to a boil, simmer for 2 minutes, add fuel, stir then turn the heat off again.

4. Place this combination into a heat-proof dish that suits your air fryer, add chicken, season with salt and pepper and steam at 350 degrees F in your fryer for 14 minutes.

5. Divide the tomatoes and the fish into plates and serve.

74.Scampi Shrimp and Chips

Preparation Time: 10 Minutes

Cooking Time: 15 Minutes

Servings: 4

Ingredients:

- 2 medium potatoes
- Salt and ground black pepper to taste
- 1 tbsp. olive oil
- 1 lb King prawns
- 1 small egg
- 5 oz. gluten-free oats

- 1 large lemon
- 1 tsp. thyme
- 1 tbsp. parsley

Directions:

1. Cut them into chunky chips after peeling the potatoes, then season with pepper and salt. Drizzle the chip with a little olive oil. Lastly, cook for 5 minutes at 360 F in an air fryer.

2. Rinse the prawns and rinse with a kitchen towel by patting them. To the chopping board, move them and season with pepper and salt.

3. Transfer the egg into a small bowl and blend until you have a beaten egg, using a fork.

4. In the blender, put 80 percent of the gluten-free oats alongside the thyme and parsley. Blend before a paste that looks like coarse breadcrumbs appear to you. Move the mixture to a medium mixing bowl.

5. In another different bowl, add the leftover 20 percent gluten-free oats.

6. Place the prawns in both the blended oats, the egg, and the blended oats.

7. Finally, put the prawns in the oats, which are not blended.

8. Place the chips on the grill pan and extract them from the air fryer.

9. Place the rest of the prawns in the air-fryer grill pan and allow them to cook at 360 F.

10. With fresh lemon juice, season the cooked prawns and chips.

11. Just serve.

75.Gambas 'Pil' with Sweet Potato

Preparation Time: 15 Minutes

Cooking Time: 20 Minutes

Servings: 3-4

Ingredients:

- 12 King prawns
- 4 garlic cloves
- 1 red chili pepper, de-seeded
- 1 shallot
- 4 tbsp. olive oil

- Smoked paprika powder

- 5 large sweet potatoes

- 2 tbsp. olive oil

- 1 tbsp. honey

- 2 tbsp. fresh rosemary, finely chopped

- 4 stalks lemongrass

- 2 limes

Directions:

1. Clean the prawns and gut them.

2. Perfect the garlic and red chili pepper, and chop the shallots.

3. To form a marinade, combine the red chili pepper, garlic, and olive oil alongside the paprika. Let the prawns marinate in the marinade for approximately 2 hours.

4. By cutting the sweet potato, make perfect slices. Using 2 tablespoons of olive oil, honey, and chopped rosemary to mix the potato slices. Inside of an air fryer, bake the potatoes at 360 F for 15 minutes.

5. Thread the prawns onto the lemongrass stalks when baking the potatoes. Increase the temperature to 390 F, and the prawn skewers are also included.

6. Allow 5 minutes to cook the mixture.

7. Serve alongside wedges of lime.

76.Fried Hot Prawns with Cocktail Sauce

Preparation Time: 5 Minutes

Cooking Time: 15 Minutes

Servings: 4

Ingredients:

- 1 tsp. chili powder

- 1 tsp. chili flakes

- ½ tsp. freshly ground black pepper

- ½ tsp. sea salt

- 8-12 fresh king prawns

For sause:

- 1 tbsp. cider or wine vinegar
- 1 tbsp. ketchup
- 3 tbsp. mayonnaise

Directions:

1. Ensure that your Air Fryer is set to 360 F.

2. Get a clean bowl and combine the spices in it.

3. Coat the prawns by tossing them in the spices mixture.

4. Transfer the spicy prawns into the air fryer basket and place the basket in the air fryer.

5. Allow the prawns to cook for 6 to 8 minutes (how long depends on the size of the prawns).

6. Get another clean bowl and make a mixture of the sauce ingredients.

7. Serve the prawns while hot alongside the cocktail sauce.

77. Crispy Air-fryer Coconut Prawns

Preparation Time: 10 Minutes

Cooking Time: 15 Minutes

Servings: 2

Ingredients:

- 1 lb fresh prawns
- 3 oz. granola
- 1 tbsp. Chinese five-spice
- 1 tbsp. mixed spice
- 1 tbsp. coriander
- Salt and ground black pepper to taste
- 1 lime rind and juice
- 2 tbsp. light coconut milk
- 3 tbsp. desiccated coconut
- 1 small egg

Directions:

1. After cleaning your prawns, lay them out on a chopping board.

2. Blend the granola in a blender until it appears like fine breadcrumbs.

3. Before removing the granola blend from the blender, add all the seasonings, lime, and coconut mix.

4. Whizz the blender around again.

5. Get a clean bowl and beat your egg in it using a fork.

6. While holding each prawn by the tail, dip it into the egg and the batter one after another.

7. After dipping all the prawns line the baking sheet at the bottom of the air fryer with your prawns.

8. Allow cooking at 360 F for 18 minutes.

9. Serve the cooked prawns.

11. King Prawns In Ham with Red Pepper Dip

Preparation Time: 10 Minutes

Cooking Time: 20 Minutes

Servings: 10

Ingredients:

- 1 large red bell pepper, halved
- 10 (frozen) king prawns, defrosted
- 5 slices of raw ham
- 1 tbsp. olive oil
- ½ tbsp. paprika
- 1 large clove garlic, crushed
- Salt to taste
- Freshly ground black pepper to taste
- Tapas forks

Directions:

1. Ensure the heating process of the air fryer to 390 F.

2. Place the bell pepper in the basket of the air fryer and let it roast for 10 minutes; extract when the skin is finely charred.

3. In a bowl, move the roasted bell pepper when covering it with an adhesive film or lid. Allow it for about 15 minutes to relax.

4. To allow you to take the black vein out, peel your prawns and make a deep incision in the back. Lengthwise, cut the ham into strips, and wrap each prawn in each slice of ham.

5. Using a thin film of olive oil to cover each parcel and transfer it into the basket. Place the basket back in the air fryer and let fry for 3 minutes. Once the prawns appear crispy and just right, withdraw.

6. Peel off the skin of the bell pepper halves while frying the prawns, and get rid of the seeds too. Then cut the pepper into bits and, besides olive oil, paprika, and garlic, purée the pieces in the blender. In a dish, pass the sauce and add pepper and salt to taste.

7. Serve in a pan alongside tapas forks the prawns in damage. A little dish of red pepper dip should be included.

78. Crispy Crabstick Crackers

Preparation Time: 10 Minutes

Cooking Time: 15 Minutes

Servings: 2-3

Ingredients:

- 1 packet Crabstick Filament, thawed
- Cooking Spray

Directions:

1. Ensure that the setting of your Air Fryer is 360 F.

2. Peel and unroll them after detaching the plastic wrapping on of crabstick filament. Finally, separate them into small pieces, which is good for thicker crackers 1/2 inch wide.

3. Spray them with a cooking spray before moving them into the frying basket.

4. Transfer the crab sticks to the air fryer in batches.

5. For 8-10 minutes, air fry each batch.

6. Remove the tray in the fourth minute and stir the crabstick crackers with the kitchen tongs, which ensures they do not stick together.

7. Adjust and allow to cool before storing them in an airtight container when air frying is completed.

79.Wasabi Crab Cakes

Preparation Time: 10 Minutes

Cooking Time: 25 Minutes

Servings: 2

Ingredients:

- 2 large egg whites
- 1 celery rib, finely chopped
- 1 medium sweet red pepper, finely chopped
- 3 green onions, finely chopped
- ¼ tsp. prepared wasabi
- 3 tbsp. reduced-fat mayonnaise
- ¼ tsp. salt
- 1/3 cup plus ½ cup dry bread crumbs, divided
- 1-1/2 cups lump crabmeat, drained
- Cooking spray

Sauce:

- ½ tsp. prepared wasabi
- 1 green onion, chopped
- 1 celery rib, chopped
- 1 tbsp. sweet pickle relish
- ¼ tsp. celery salt
- 1/3 cup reduced-fat mayonnaise

Directions:

1. Make sure the Air Fryer is preheated to 375 F and that the basket of the air fryer is sprayed with cooking spray.

2. Get a bowl and, along with 1/3 cup breadcrumbs, make a mixture of the first seven ingredients. Fold in the crab softly.

3. Take a shallow bowl and place in the remaining bread crumbs. Then add the bowl of heaping tablespoonful of crab mixture. Coat and shape the crumbs into 3/4-inch-thick patties.

4. If required, you should operate in samples batch of crab cakes should be arranged to form a single layer in the air fryer basket.

5. Just cook with cooking spray after spritzing the crab cakes.

6. It should take about 8 to 12 minutes to cook, or until the cakes turn golden brown. Turn the cakes halfway through heating, then spritz again with extra cooking oil.

7. Withdraw and keep warm once cooked.

8. For the other batches, do the same.

9. Place the sauce ingredients in your food processor while cooking the cakes, and blend to the preferred consistency.

10. In addition to the dipping sauce, serve fried crabs while warm.

80.Flourless Truly Crispy Calamari Rings

Preparation Time: 05 Minutes

Cooking Time: 10 Minutes

Servings: 2

Ingredients:

- 1 oz. calamari
- 1 cup gluten-free oats
- 1 large egg, beaten
- 1 tbsp. paprika
- 1 tsp. parsley
- 1 small lemon juice and rind
- Salt and ground black pepper to taste

Directions:

1. Ensure that your Air Fryer is preheated to 360 F.

2. Slice your calamari thinly to produce small rings of calamari.

3. Using a food processor or a blender, blend your oats until you have a consistency that looks like that of fine breadcrumbs.

4. Transfer the beaten egg to a separate bowl and the oats to another bowl.

5. Mix the oats with paprika and parsley.

6. Get a chopping board, and coat your calamari rings on it using salt, lemon, and pepper.

7. Your hands may be sticky; thus, ensure you rub them in the oats.

8. Transfer the calamari rings into the oats first, then into the egg, then the oats, why ensuring that they are thoroughly coated at each stage.

9. Get rid of any excess oats and transfer the rings into the baking mat of your air fryer.

10. Allow cooking for 8 minutes at 360 F.

11. Serve!

81.Scallops Wrapped in Bacon

Preparation Time: 10 Minutes

Cooking Time: 15 Minutes

Servings: 4

Ingredients:

- 8 scallops
- 8 bacon slices
- Toothpicks

Directions:

1. Wrap the bacon over the scallop.

2. Hold it in place with a toothpick.

3. Set your air fryer to 360 F and air fry the bacon.

4. Withdraw after 18 minutes or when a beautiful golden brown color is observed.

82.Tilapia Fillet with Vegetables
Preparation Time: 20 Minutes

Cooking Time: 40 Minutes

Servings: 2

Ingredients:

- 2 tilapia fillets Mushrooms to taste
- 1 broccoli
- 1 sweet potato

- 1 carrot Seasoning to taste

Directions:

1. Grill and sauté the mushrooms in the oil.

2. Cut the vegetables, season and place on a baking sheet and close with laminated paper.

3. Baked it in the fryer at 4000F for 25 minutes.

4. Make a beautiful dish and have a good appetite.

83.Shrimps in the Pumpkin
Preparation Time: 10 Minutes

Cooking Time: 30 Minutes

Servings: 4

Ingredients:

- 2 ¼ lb of medium shrimp
- 4 tbsp. of olive oil
- 2 cloves of garlic
- 1 onion
- 5 seedless tomatoes, Salt and black pepper to taste.
- 1 can of cream without serum
- ½ lb of cream cheese
- 1 strawberry
- green aroma to taste
- 3 tbsp. of tomato sauce

Directions:

1. Remove the top and the strawberry seeds.

2. Wash and seal in foil and bake at 360 ° F for 45 minutes in an air fryer.

3. Heat the oil and sauté the garlic and onion in a saucepan, add the shrimp, and cook for 5 minutes.

4. Stir in the diced tomatoes, salt, pepper and tomato sauce.

5. Turn the heat off and apply the green smell and cream.

6. Mix well, and then apply the curd.

7. Place the strawberry inside a bit of curd and pour the shrimp cream.

84.Shrimp Strogonoff

Preparation Time: 10 Minutes

Cooking Time: 15 Minutes

Servings: 2-4

Ingredients:

- 1 tbsp. butter 1 medium
- Onion grated
- 1 lb of medium clean shrimp
- Salt and pepper
- 4 tbsp. of brandy
- 3 ½ oz. minced pickled mushrooms
- 3 tbsp. of tomato sauce
- 1 tbsp. of mustard
- 1 can of cream set aside.

Directions:

1. Make the shrimp clean. Remove the peels and use water and lemon to wash them very well.

2. Heat the onion butter and brown it. Season with salt and pepper, remove from the heat and blend with the shrimp and stir well.

3. Put the fryer in the air for 5 minutes at 3200F.

4. In a shell, heat the cognac until it catches fire. Then spill it over the burning shrimp.

5. Add the mushroom, tomato sauce, mustard and cook for about 5 minutes in an air fryer.

6. Add the milk before serving, stir well and steam without boiling. 7. Use white rice and straw potatoes to eat the stroganoff.

85.Pumpkin Shrimp with Catupiry

Preparation Time: 20 Minutes

Cooking Time: 30 Minutes

Servings: 2-4

Ingredients:

- 1 large strawberry
- 2 ¼ lb of medium shrimp
- 1 pot of catupiry
- 1 glass of palm heart
- 1 bottle of coconut milk Salt Chile
- 1 grated onion
- 2 cloves of garlic
- 2 chopped seedless tomatoes
- 1 tbsp. of wheat flour dessert

Directions:

1. Remove the cap of the strawberry and all the seeds then. Spray salt on the interior after cleaning. Wrap the aluminum foil around the whole strawberry. Bake at 4000F in an air-fryer for 45 minutes. Set back, but before using a spoon, add some strawberry slices to the stew.

2. In the fat, cook the onion and garlic. Then she took out the tomatoes and strawberry slices, leaving them too steep for 10 minutes. Attach the sliced palm kernel and then the shrimp that you shouldn't cook for more than 10 minutes, so it's going to be completely hard if you cook it longer. To make it slightly thick, add the coconut milk and 1 tablespoon of flour dissolved in water. And apply half the catupiry box to the prepared stir fry and turn off, mixing it well into the stir fry and salt.

3. Take catupiry balls with your hands with the strawberry still hot and put them on the bottom and sides (the catupiry must be very cold to stick more easily).

4. Pour in the strawberry with the hot stir fry and eat.

5. Put in parsley or coriander to taste (it depends on the flavor of each one).

86.Fricassee of Jamila Shrimps
Preparation Time: 15 Minutes

Cooking Time: 40 Minutes

Servings: 2-5

Ingredients:

- 2 ¼ lb clean shrimp

- Salt and pepper to taste olive oil

- 1 large grated onion Chopped garlic

- 3 tomatoes, chopped parsley and chives

- 1 can of vegetable

- 1 can of sour cream

- 1 can of corn grated

- cheese to taste

- 2 glasses of curd

- ½ lb mozzarella cheese

- potato sticks

Directions:

1. Wash the shrimp and season with salt, pepper and lemon. Allow time for the seasoning to soak in.

2. Sauté the grated onion, minced garlic, tomatoes, parsley, and chives in olive oil.

3. Add the shrimp and the garden. Mix and cook for about 5 minutes or until shrimp are pink. Reserve.

4. Whisk the corn with sour cream and grated cheese in a blender.

5. Spread the creamy curd, shrimp sauce on a plate, and then pour the whipped cream on top.

6. Cover with mozzarella.

7. Take to the air fryer to brown at 3600F for 30 minutes.

8. Serve hot with white rice and straw potatoes.

87.Fried Beach Shrimps
Preparation Time: 5 Minutes

Cooking Time: 15 Minutes

Servings: 2-4

Ingredients:

- 2 ¼ lb of clean and washed gray shrimp

- ½ lemon Salt 1

- ½ tbsp. of flour

- 2 garlic cloves, squeezed

Directions:

1. Season shrimp (must be very dry) with salt, lemon, and squeezed garlic.

2. Sprinkle the flour and mix well.

3. Take to the air fryer at 3600F for 15 minutes and fry until golden. Serve well with a leafy salad and white rice.

88.Fried Shrimp without Flour

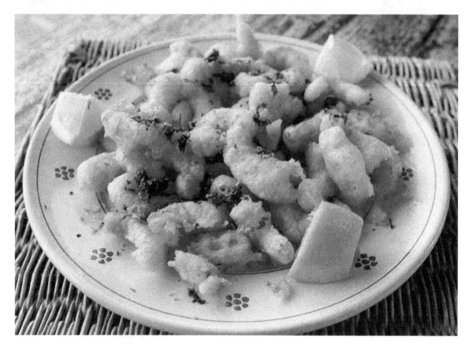

Preparation Time: 5 Minutes

Cooking Time: 10 Minutes

Servings: 2

Ingredients:

- ½ lb small shrimp without shell
- 2 tbsp. of olive oil
- 2 garlic cloves, crushed
- ½ large onion, chopped
- 2 tbsp. soy sauce salt to taste black pepper to taste

Directions:

1. In a pan, add a little olive oil, crushed garlic, and onion, marinate for 5 minutes.

2. Add the shrimp, salt, black pepper, and soy sauce.

3. Take to the air fryer at 3600 F. Let it cook for 10 minutes.

4. Let shrimp fry until golden brown, then sprinkle with Parmesan cheese.

5. Parsley to taste grated fresh parmesan cheese to taste

89.Shrimps with Garlic and Oil

Preparation Time: 10 Minutes

Cooking Time: 15 Minutes

Servings: 4-6

Ingredients:

- 3 lbs. medium shrimp
- 10 cloves of garlic
- Salt to taste
- Olive oil to taste

Directions:

1. Wash the shrimp in the shell, with the head removed.

2. Peel the cloves of garlic, and cut them in half.

3. Fry the garlic in the oil well (well done).

4. Place the shrimp in a saucepan and sprinkle it with some salt.

5. Take it to the 3200F air fryer for 5 minutes.

6. Place the oil in a bowl with the garlic and pour it over it.

7. Serve with beer with snow.

90.Breaded Prawns

Preparation Time: 5 Minutes

Cooking Time: 15 Minutes

Servings: 1-2

Ingredients:

- 12 large prawns

- 3 tablespoons butter, melted
- 6 eggs Wheat flour to the point Salt to taste
- 1 tbsp. of virgin olive oil

Directions:

1. Cook the prawns in the air fryer at 3200F, being careful not to cook them for about 10 minutes. Remove.

2. Then peel the prawns and place them in the melted butter, resting.

3. Separate the whites from the yolks of the 6 eggs, beating the whites in the snow, then add the wheat flour until it sighs, season with salt and the spoon of oil.

4. Then, place the prawns in this pasta and with a spoon, remove each shrimp, accompanied by a little pasta.

5. Put back in the air fryer for 5 minutes.

91. Vegetable Supreme Pan Pizza

Preparation Time: 15 Minutes

Cooking Time: 30 Minutes

Servings: 3

Ingredients:

- 8 slice White Onion
- 12 slice Tomato
- 2 tablespoon olive oil
- 3/2 cup shredded mozzarella
- 8 Cremini mushrooms
- 1/2 green pepper
- 4 tablespoon Pesto
- 1 Pizza Dough
- 1 cup spinach

Directions:

1. Roll the pizza dough halves until they each meet the size of the Air Flow racks.

2. Grease all sides of each dough lightly with olive oil.

3. On a rack, put each pizza. Place the racks on the electric fryer's upper and lower shelves.

4. Then press the power button and the cooking time to 13 minutes by pressing the French Fries button (400° F).

5. Flip the dough onto the top shelf after 5 minutes and switch the racks.

6. Switch the dough on to the top shelf after 4 minutes.

7. Take both racks out and drizzle the toppings with the pizzas.

8. Place the racks on the electric fryer's upper and lower shelves.

9. Then push the power button and the cooking time to 7 minutes by pressing the French Fries button (400° F).

10. Rotate the pizzas after 4 minutes.

11. If the pizzas are done, let them rest before cutting them for 4 minutes.

92. Pignoli Cookies

Preparation Time: 15 Minutes

Cooking Time: 25 Minutes

Servings: 36

Ingredients:

- 2 cup pine nuts
- 4 large egg whites
- 1 cup confectioners' sugar
- 1/2 cup sugar
- 10-ounce almond paste

Directions:

1. In a bowl, whisk the almond paste and sugar together until just mixed.

2. Through the almond mixture, add 2 egg whites.

3. Add the confectioner's sugar to the almond mixture gradually and blend well to form a dough.

4. Until the whites are foamy, pound the remaining two egg whites in a separate bowl.

5. To prevent the dough from sticking to your fingers, dip your fingers in the flour. Shape 1 inch into the dough. In the egg whites, dip the balls and coat each ball with the pine nuts.

6. Place the balls and flatten each ball gently on two parchment-lined Air Flow Racks.

7. On the bottom and middle shelves of the appliance, place the racks.

8. Press the power button, the cooking temperature is lowered to 325 ° F, and the cooking time is increased to 18 minutes. Switch racks in the middle of cooking time (9 minutes).

93. Jam Filled Buttermilk Scones

Preparation Time: 15 Minutes

Cooking Time: 25 Minutes

Servings: 6

Ingredients:

- 2¼ cup flour
- 1 teaspoon salt
- 1/4 cup sugar
- 2 teaspoon Baking Powder
- 12 tablespoon butter
- 2 large eggs
- 1/3 cup buttermilk
- 1 teaspoon Vanilla Extract
- 1/2 cup strawberry jams
- 2 tablespoon demerara sugar

Directions:

1. In a container, mix the baking powder, flour, sugar and salt together.

2. Using the wider holes on a box grater, grind the butter into the dish.

3. Combine the cup with the ingredients.

4. To complete the dough, whisk together the patted eggs, vanilla, and buttermilk into the bowl.

5. Break the dough in two, form each half of the dough into a disc, cover the discs with plastic wrap and put them in the fridge for 60 minutes.

6. Using a fresh sheet of plastic wrap to position a disc. Roll the disc to a thickness of 1/2 inch.

7. Spread the jam on the disk leaving a ½ in. scab around the edges.

8. Roll the other disc to 1/2-inch thickness into another layer of plastic wrap.

9. Place the second discover the first disc and press softly to secure the discs' edges.

10. Made into eight wedges with the dough.

11. On two parchment-lined Air Flow shelves, put shims. Brush the wedges with the buttermilk generously and dust with the Demerara sugar. Place the racks on the appliance's bottom and center shelves.

12. Press the power button to raise the cooking temperature to 375 degrees F and simmer for 18 minutes. After 10 mins, rotate the shelves.

94. Chicken Milanese
Preparation Time: 10 Minutes

Cooking Time: 20 Minutes

Servings: 3

Ingredients:

- 4 chicken cutlets
- 2 tablespoon Extra Virgin Olive Oil
- Juice of 1/2 lemon
- Shaved parmesan for garnish
- 2 cup panko breadcrumbs
- 2 eggs, beaten
- 1 teaspoon Garlic powder
- 1 beefsteak tomato, diced
- Salt and black pepper, divided
- 3 cup arugula
- 1/4 cup parmesan, grated
- 1 teaspoon White wine vinegar

Directions:

1. Bring the panko breadcrumbs, parmesan, and garlic powder together in a dish.

2. With salt and pepper, softly season the chicken cutlets.

3. In a separate bowl, add the eggs.

4. Through the egg, drop the cutlets. Then coat the panko mixture with it.

5. On the Air Flow Racks, position the cutlets

6. Click the Button for Steaks/Chops (370°F). To start the cooking cycle, reduce the cooking time to 15 minutes.

7. Prepare the salad when the chicken is preparing food: stir in the lemon juice, olive oil, vinegar and a pinch of salt and pepper in a container.

8. Use the dressing to add the arugula and coat.

9. Place the chicken on a plate when the chicken is done eating and top with the chopped tomato and the arugula salad, and top with the shaved Parmesan.

95. White Pizza
Preparation Time: 15 Minutes

Cooking Time: 25 Minutes

Servings: 1

Ingredients:

- 2 clove garlic, thinly sliced
- 1 thin-crust pizza dough
- 9 slice fresh mozzarella
- 1 teaspoon red pepper flakes
- 1/4 cup ricotta cheese
- 2 tablespoon extra-virgin olive oil, divided

Directions:

1. Use 1 tablespoon of olive oil to rub the pizza dough. To suit on an Air Flow rack, roll the pizza dough out.

2. Put the pizza on the rack and slide it onto the Air Fryer oven center shelf.

3. Press the control button and then the (400 ° F / 200 ° C) French Fries button. To begin the cooking cycle, you manually set the cooking time to 10 minutes. Turn the dough over halfway through the cooking time (5 minutes).

4. From the Air Fryer oven, remove the crust.

5. Drizzle the ricotta, mozzarella, garlic and red pepper flakes with the crust. Bring the pizza back to the Power Air Fryer oven.

6. Press the control button and then the (400 ° F / 200 ° C) French Fries button. To begin the cooking cycle, you manually set the cooking time to 6 minutes. Cook until you've melted the cheese.

7. One teaspoon Drizzle. Before eating, place olive oil on the pizza.

96. Cheddar Biscuits
Preparation Time: 10 Minutes

Cooking Time: 30 Minutes

Servings: 16

Ingredients:

- 3/4 cup buttermilk
- 1/2 teaspoon seafood seasoning
- 1/2 cup scallions, chopped
- 1/4 teaspoon Cayenne powder
- 2 cup flour
- 1 stick butter
- 2 teaspoon Baking Powder
- 3/2 cup cheddar, shredded

Directions:

1. In a bowl, combine the flour and butter until it is pea-size.

2. Add the remaining ingredients and whisk.

3. Divide into 16 balls and place in an Air Flow Rack.

4. Press the baking button. Reduce the timer to 15 minutes to start the cook cycle.

5. Serve.

97. Maryland Crab Cakes
Preparation Time: 10 Minutes

Cooking Time: 20 Minutes

Servings: 5

Ingredients:

- 1 teaspoon salt
- 1 cup cracker crumbs
- 1 pound Lump crab meat
- 1 pinch salt and pepper to season
- 2 tablespoon fresh parsley, chopped
- 1 teaspoon seafood seasoning
- 1/2 teaspoon ground black pepper
- 1/4 cup scallions, finely chopped
- 1 tablespoon sweet chili sauce
- 1 teaspoon garlic, minced
- 1 cup mayonnaise
- 1 tablespoon sweet pickle relish
- 1/4 cup Celery, diced
- 1 tablespoon Lemon juice
- 1 tablespoon Thai chili sauce

Directions:

1. In a large bowl, bring together all the breadcrumb ingredients except the crabmeat and cookie crumbs.

2. Gently mix the crab meat and 1/4 cup of the cracker crumbs.

3. Spread the remaining crumbs out on a work surface.

4. Form 12 equal-sized balls with crab mixture.

5. Place the balls on top of the crumbs to coat evenly and press gently to make a patty.

6. Place in a refrigerator for 20 minutes.

7. Place the crab cakes on the Air Flow racks.

8. Press the Steaks / Chops button. Reduce the timer to 20 minutes to begin the cook cycle.

9. While the crab cakes are cooking, prepare the dipping sauce: combine all the ingredients and season with salt and pepper.

10. Serve hot crab cakes with dipping sauce.

98. Pepperoni Stuffed Mozzarella Patties
Preparation Time: 15 Minutes

Cooking Time: 30 Minutes

Servings: 12

Ingredients:

- 2 cup seasoned Italian breadcrumbs
- 24 slice pepperonis
- 1-pound whole milk mozzarella
- 4 eggs beaten

Directions:

1. Cut a mozzarella block into 1/4-inch slices. Chop each slice in half.

2. Place two pepperoni slices over the middle of the slices.

3. Create a cheese sandwich with the rest of the mozzarella halves and press tightly to seal.

4. Prepare a dredging station using flour, eggs and breadcrumbs. Dip each mozzarella sandwich in the flour, then the egg, then the breadcrumbs. Once more, dip each sandwich back into the egg and then into the breadcrumbs.

5. Sprinkle patties with cooking spray.

6. Cook sandwiches in the Air Fryer Oven at 400 degrees F for 6 minutes, turning patties midway through cooking.

99. Corned Beef and Cabbage Egg Rolls
Preparation Time: 10 Minutes

Cooking Time: 20 Minutes

Servings: 12

Ingredients:

- 3/2 cup stewed cabbage
- 12 egg roll wrappers
- 3/4-pound corned beef, shredded
- Spicy Mustard

Directions:

1. Working with one egg roll wrapper at a time, position the wrap with one corner of the wrap facing you.

2. Use about 2 tablespoons of minced corned beef to create a small log in the middle of the wrapper. Top the corned beef with 1 tablespoon shredded cabbage. Roll the corner of the egg roll wrapper over the filling and cautiously fold in the wrapper to form an airtight seal.

3. Scrub the rest of the edges of the wrapper with water. Fold each side of the wrap and then roll the egg roll to seal. Redo until all the meat and cabbage are gone.

4. Position the egg rolls on an Air Flow rack. Spray muffins with cooking spray. Slide the rack onto the center shelf of the Air Fryer oven. Press the French fry's button (400°F), set the cooking time to 7 minutes and cook until golden brown.

5. When the egg rolls are done, serve them warm with spicy mustard.

100. Fish Tacos
Preparation Time: 10 Minutes

Cooking Time: 30 Minutes

Servings: 6

Ingredients:

- 6 flour tortillas
- 1 cup coleslaw
- 1 cup panko breadcrumbs
- 1/2 cup salsa
- 1/2 cup guacamole
- 1 cup flour
- 3/2 cup seltzer water, cold

- 2 tablespoon cilantros, chopped

- 1 lemon, cut into wedges

- 10-ounce cod filet

- 1 teaspoon ground white pepper

- 1 tablespoon Cornstarch

- Salt, to taste, divided

Directions:

Tempura Batter:

1. In a bowl, bring together the flour, cornstarch and salt.

2. Mix in the cold seltzer.

3. Mix all the ingredients until consistency is attained.

Taco:

1. Cut the cod fillet into long 2-oz. pieces and season with salt and white pepper.

2. In a skillet: Add the panko breadcrumbs. Dip each piece of cod in the tempura batter. Next, dredge the cod in the panko breadcrumbs.

3. Position the breaded cod on the Air Flow racks. Slide racks into Power Air Fryer oven.

4. Set the appliance to the French fries setting (400°F). Set the cooking time to 10 minutes.

5. Midway through the cook cycle, turn the fish sticks.

6. Once the cooking time is over, remove the fish rods.

7. Spread the guacamole on a tortilla. Place a fish stick on the tortilla and top with some coleslaw, salsa, and a dash of lemon. Top with chopped cilantro.

8. Repeat until all ingredients are used up.

9. Fold the tacos before eating.

Conclusion

You already know that if you have an air fryer, it's a futuristic gadget designed to save time and make you live easier. You'll be excited to hear about how soon you'll be addicted to use your air fryer to cook almost every meal if you've still not taken the jump. Don't think much and kick start a healthy living. This book will provide you with lots of amazing recipes to make using your air fryer.

The Affordable Air Fryer Cookbook

The Ultimate Guide with 100 Quick and Delicious Affordable Recipes for beginners

By Marisa Smith

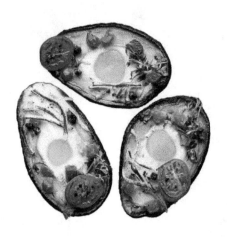

Introduction

We all love the deep-fried food taste, but not the calories or hassle of frying in too much fat. To solve this issue, the Air fryer was designed as its revolutionary nature allows you to cook food while frying with one or two tablespoons of oil and remove extra fat from the meal. This recipe book includes some of the amazing recipes that your Air fryer can prepare. From French fries to spring rolls and even soufflés, the choices are limitless!

Air Fryer Recipes

1. Chewy Breakfast Brownies

Total time: 40 min

Prep time: 10 min

Cook time: 30 min

Yield: 9 servings

Ingredients:

- 1 egg
- 2 tbsp. cocoa powder
- 1 tsp. vanilla
- 1 1/4 cup milk
- 1/2 cup applesauce
- 1/4 cup brown sugar
- 2 1/4 cup quick oats

Directions:

1. Spray and set aside a 9*9-inch baking dish with cooking spray.

2. Insert a rack of wire in rack position 6. Pick bake, set temperature to 350 f, 30-minute timer. To preheat the oven, press start.

3. Mix brown sugar, cocoa powder, and oats together in a big cup.

4. Add wet ingredients: blend until well mixed.

5. Pour the baking dish with the mixture and spread it properly.

6. Place foil on the baking dish and bake for 15 minutes. After 15 minutes, remove the cover and bake for 15 more minutes.

7. Enjoy and serve.

2.Peach Banana Baked Oatmeal

Total time: 45 min

Prep time: 10 min

Cook time: 35 min

Yield: 5 servings

Ingredients:

- Two eggs
- 1 tsp. vanilla
- 1 1/2 cups milk
- 1/2 tsp. cinnamon
- 3/4 tsp. baking powder
- 1/4 cup ground flax seed
- 2 1/2 cups steel-cut oats
- 2 bananas, sliced
- 1 peach, sliced
- 1/2 tsp. salt

Directions:

1. Spray an 8*8-inch baking dish with cooking spray and set aside.
2. Insert wire rack in rack position 6. Select bake, set temperature 350 f, timer for 35 minutes. Press start to preheat the oven.
3. Add all ingredients except one banana into the mixing bowl and mix until well combined.
4. Pour mixture into the baking dish and spread well. Spread the remaining 1 banana slices on top and bake for 35 minutes.
5. Serv e and enjoy.

3.Healthy Poppy seed Baked Oatmeal

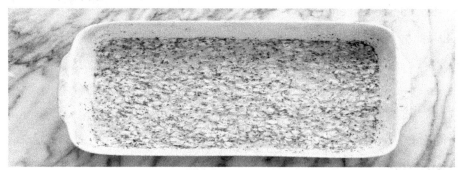

Total time: 35 min

Prep time: 10 min

Cook time: 25 min

Yield: 8 servings

Ingredients:

- 3 eggs
- 1 tbsp. poppy seeds
- 1 tsp. baking powder
- 1 tsp. vanilla
- 1 tsp. lemon zest
- 1/4 cup lemon juice
- 1/4 cup honey
- 2 cups almond milk
- 3 cups rolled oats
- 1/4 tsp. salt

Directions:

1. Spray a baking dish with cooking spray and set it aside.

2. Insert wire rack in rack position 6. Select bake, set temperature 350 f, timer for 25 minutes. Press start to preheat the oven.

3. In a large bowl, mix together all ingredients: until well combined.

4. Pour mixture into the baking dish and spread well, and bake for 25 minutes.

5. Serve and enjoy.

4.Healthy Berry Baked Oatmeal

Total time: 30 min

Prep time: 10 min

Cook time: 20 min

Yield: 4 servings

Ingredients:

- 1 egg
- 1 cup blueberries
- 1/2 cup blackberries
- 1/2 cup strawberries, sliced
- 1/4 cup maple syrup
- 1 1/2 cups milk
- 1 1/2 tsp. baking powder
- 2 cups old fashioned oats
- 1/2 tsp. salt

Directions:

1. Spray with cooking spray on a baking dish and put aside.

2. Insert a rack of wire in rack position 6. Pick bake, set temperature to 375 f, 20 minute timer. To preheat the oven, press start.

3. Blend together the peas, salt and baking powder in a mixing cup. Stir well and Mix vanilla, egg, maple syrup, and tea.

4. Add berries and blend well with them. Into the baking bowl, add the mixture and bake for 20 minutes.

5. Enjoy and serve.

5.Apple Oatmeal Bars

Total time: 35 min

Prep time: 10 min

Cook time: 25 min

Yield: 12 servings

Ingredients:

- 2 eggs
- 2 tbsp. butter
- 2 tsp. baking powder
- 2 cups apple, chopped
- 3 cups old fashioned oats
- Pinch of salt
- 1/2 cup honey
- 1 tbsp. vanilla
- 1 cup milk
- 1 tbsp. cinnamon

Directions:

1. Spray a 9*13-inch baking dish with cooking spray and set aside.
2. Insert wire rack in rack position 6. Select bake, set temperature 375 f, timer for 25 minutes. Press start to preheat the oven.
3. In a mixing bowl, mix together dry ingredients.
4. In a separate bowl, whisk together wet ingredients. Pour wet ingredient mixture into the dry mixture and mix well.
5. Pour mixture into the baking dish and bake for 25 minutes.
6. Slice and serve.

6.Walnut Banana Bread

Prep time: 10 minutes

Cook time: 50 minutes

Yield: 10 servings

Ingredients:

- 3 eggs
- 1 tsp. baking soda
- 4 tbsp. olive oil
- 1/2 cup walnuts, chopped
- 2 cups almond flour
- 3 bananas

Directions:

1. Grease loaf pan with butter and set aside.
2. Insert wire rack in rack position 6. Select bake, set temperature 350 f, timer for 50 minutes. Press start to preheat the oven.
3. Add all ingredients into the food processor and process until combined.
4. Pour batter into the prepared loaf pan and bake for 50 minutes.
5. Slices and serve.

7.Cinnamon Zucchini Bread

Total time: 1 hour 10 min

Prep time: 10 min

Cook time: 60 min

Yield: 12 servings

Ingredients:

- 3 eggs
- 1/2 tsp. nutmeg
- 1 1/2 tsp. baking powder
- 1 1/2 tsp. erythritol
- 2 1/2 cups almond flour
- 1 tsp. vanilla

- 1/2 cup walnuts, chopped
- 1 cup zucchini, grated & squeeze out all liquid
- 1/4 tsp. ground ginger
- 1 tsp. cinnamon
- 1/2 cup olive oil
- 1/2 tsp. salt

Directions:

1. Grease loaf pan with butter and set aside.
2. Insert wire rack in rack position 6. Select bake, set temperature 350 f, timer for 60 minutes. Press start to preheat the oven.
3. In a bowl, whisk eggs, vanilla, and oil. Set aside.
4. In a separate bowl, mix together almond flour, ginger, cinnamon, nutmeg, baking powder, salt, and sweetener. Set aside.
5. Add grated zucchini into the egg mixture and stir well.
6. Add dry ingredients into the egg mixture and stir to combine.
7. Pour batter into the loaf pan and bake for 60 minutes.
8. Slices and serve.

8. Italian Breakfast Bread

Total time: 60 min

Prep time: 10 min

Cook time: 50 min

Yield: 10 servings

Ingredients:

- 1/2 cup black olives, chopped
- 5 sun-dried tomatoes, chopped
- 2 tbsp. psyllium husk powder
- 5 egg whites
- 2 egg yolks
- 4 tbsp. coconut oil

- 2 cups flaxseed flour
- 2 tbsp. apple cider vinegar
- 1 tbsp. thyme, dried
- 1 tbsp. oregano, dried
- 2 1/2 oz. feta cheese
- 1 tbsp. baking powder
- 1/2 cup boiling water
- 1/2 tsp. salt

Directions:

1. Grease loaf pan with butter and set aside.
2. Insert wire rack in rack position 6. Select bake, set temperature 350 f, timer for 50 minutes. Press start to preheat the oven.
3. In a bowl, mix together psyllium husk powder, baking powder, and flaxseed.
4. Add oil and eggs and stir to combine. Add vinegar and stir well.
5. Add boiling water and stir to combine.
6. Add tomatoes, olives, and feta cheese. Mix well.
7. Pour batter into the loaf pan and bake for 50 minutes.
8. Sliced and serve.

9.Coconut Zucchini Bread

Total time: 55 min

Prep time: 10 min

Cook time: 45 min

Yield: 12 servings

Ingredients:

- 1 banana, mashed
- 1 tsp. stevia
- 4 eggs
- 1/2 cup coconut flour

- 1 tbsp. coconut oil
- 1 cup zucchini, shredded and squeeze out all liquid
- 1/2 cup walnuts, chopped
- 1 tbsp. cinnamon
- 3/4 tsp. baking soda
- 1/2 tsp. salt
- 1 tsp. apple cider vinegar
- 1/2 tsp. nutmeg

Directions:

1. Grease the loaf pan and set it aside with butter.
2. Wire rack insertion at rack position 6. Pick bake, set temperature to 350 f, 45 minute timer. To preheat the oven, press start.
3. Whisk the egg, banana, oil and stevia together in a big mug.
4. Stir well and add all the dried ingredients, vinegar, and zucchini. Combine the walnuts and stir.
5. Through the loaf tin, add the batter and bake for 45 minutes.
6. Slicing and cooking.

10.Protein Banana Bread

Total time: 1 hour 20 min

Prep time: 10 min

Cook time: 1 hour 10 min

Yield: 16 servings

Ingredients:

- 3 eggs
- 1/3 cup coconut flour
- 1/2 cup swerve
- 2 cups almond flour
- 1/2 cup ground chia seed

- 1/2 tsp. vanilla extract
- 4 tbsp. butter, melted
- 3/4 cup almond milk
- 1 tbsp. baking powder
- 1/3 cup protein powder
- 1/2 cup water
- 1/2 tsp. salt

Directions:

1. Grease the loaf pan and set it aside with butter.
2. Wire rack insertion at rack position 6. Bake selection, set temperature 325 f, 1 hour 10 minutes timer. To preheat the oven, press start.
3. Whisk the chia seed and 1/2 cup of water together in a small dish. Only put aside.
4. Mix the almond flour, baking powder, protein powder, coconut flour, sweetener, and salt together in a big cup.
5. Mix eggs, sugar, blend of chia seeds, vanilla extract and butter until well mixed.
6. In the prepared loaf tin, add the batter and bake for 1 hour and 10 minutes.
7. Slicing and serving

11.Easy Kale Muffins

Total time: 40 min

Prep time: 10 min

Cook time: 30 min

Yield: 8 servings

Ingredients:

- 6 eggs
- 1/2 cup milk
- 1/4 cup chives, chopped

- 1 cup kale, chopped
- Pepper
- Salt

Directions:

4. Spray 8 cups muffin pan with cooking spray and set aside.

5. Insert wire rack in rack position 6. Select bake, set temperature 350 f, timer for 30 minutes. Press start to preheat the oven.

6. Add all ingredients into the mixing bowl and whisk well.

7. Pour mixture into the prepared muffin pan and bake for 30 minutes.

8. Serve and enjoy.

12.Mouthwatering Shredded BBQ Roast

Total time: 40 min

Prep time: 10 min

Cook time: 30 min

Yield: 8 servings

Ingredients:

- 4 lbs. Pork roast
- 1 tsp. Garlic powder
- Salt and pepper to taste
- 1/2 cup water
- 2 can (11 oz.) Of barbecue sauce, keno unsweetened

Directions:

1. Season the pork with garlic powder, salt and pepper, place in your instant pot.

2. Pour water and lock lid into place; set on the meat/stew, the high-pressure setting for 30 minutes.

3. When ready, use quick release - turn the valve from sealing to venting to release the pressure.

4. Remove pork in a bowl, and with two forks, shred the meat.

5. Pour BBQ sauce and stir to combine well.

6. Serve.

13.Sour and Spicy Spareribs

Total time: 50 min

Prep time: 15 min

Cook time: 35 min

Yield: 10 servings

Ingredients:

- 5 lbs. Spare spareribs
- Salt and pepper to taste
- 2 tbsp. Of tallow
- 1/2 cup coconut amines (from coconut sap)
- 1/2 cup vinegar
- 2 tbsp. Worcestershire sauce, to taste
- 1 tsp. Chili powder
- 1 tsp. Garlic powder
- 1 tsp. Celery seeds

Directions:

1. Break into similar parts the rack of ribs.
2. Season the spareribs on both sides with salt and ground pepper.
3. In your instant pot, add tallow and put the spareribs.
4. Mix all the remaining ingredients in a cup and spill over the spareribs.
5. Click the lid in place and set it to heat for 35 minutes on the manual setting.
6. Click "cancel" as the timer beeps, then flip the natural release gently for 20 minutes.
7. Open the cover and put the ribs on a serving tray.
8. Serve it hot.

14. Tender Pork Shoulder with Hot Peppers

Prep time: 10 minutes

Cook time: 30 minutes

Yield: 8 servings

Ingredients:

- 3 lbs. Pork shoulder boneless
- Salt and ground black pepper to taste
- 3 tbsp. Of olive oil
- 1 large onion, chopped
- 2 cloves garlic minced
- 2 - 3 chili peppers, chopped
- 1 tsp. Ground coriander
- 1 tsp. ground cumin
- 1 ½ cups of bone broth (preferably homemade)
- 1/2 cup water

Directions:

1. Season the salt and the pork meat with pepper.
2. Switch the instant pot on and press the button to sauté. When the term 'heat' appears on the show, add the oil and sauté for around 5 minutes with the onions and garlic.
3. Add the pork and cook on both sides for 1 - 2 minutes; turn off the sauté button.
4. In an instant kettle, add all the remaining ingredients.
5. Click the lid in place and set it on high heat for 30 minutes on the meat/stew level.
6. Click "cancel" as the timer beeps, then flip the natural release button gently for 15 minutes. Serve it warm.

15. Braised Sour Pork Filet

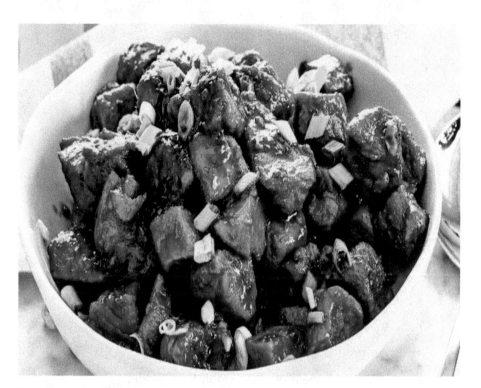

Prep time: 10 minutes

Cook time: 8 hours

Yield: 6 servings

Ingredients:

- 1/2 tsp. Of dry thyme
- 1/2 tsp. Of sage
- Salt and ground black pepper to taste
- 2 tabs of olive oil
- 3 lbs. Of pork fillet
- 1/3 cup of shallots (chopped)
- Three cloves of garlic (minced)
- 3/4 cup of bone broth
- 1/3 cup of apple cider vinegar

Directions:

1. Combine the thyme, sage, salt and black ground pepper in a shallow cup.

2. Rub the pork generously on both edges.

3. In a large frying pan, heat the olive oil and cook the pork for 2 - 3 minutes.

4. Place the pork and add the shallots and garlic in your crockpot.

5. Sprinkle with broth and apple cider vinegar/juice.

6. Cover and simmer for 8 hours on slow heat or 4-5 hours on high heat.

7. Change the salt and pepper, slice and serve with cooking juice and cut the pork from the pan.

16.Pork with Anise and Cumin Stir-Fry

Total time: 35 min

Prep time: 5 min

Cook time: 30 min

Yield: 4 servings

Ingredients:

- 2 tbsp. Lard
- 2 spring onions finely chopped (only green part)
- 2 cloves garlic, finely chopped
- 2 lbs. Pork loin, boneless, cut into cubes
- Sea salt and black ground pepper to taste
- 1 green bell pepper (cut into thin strips)
- 1/2 cup water
- 1/2 tsp. Dill seeds
- 1/2 anise seeds
- 1/2 tsp. Cumin

Directions:

1. Heat the lard n a large frying pot over medium-high heat.

2. Sauté the spring onions and garlic with a pinch of salt for 3 - 4 minutes.

3. Add the pork and simmer for about 5 - 6 minutes.

4. Add all remaining ingredients: and stir well.

5. Cover and let simmer for 15 - 20 minutes

6. Taste and adjust seasoning to taste.

7. Serve!

17.Baked Meatballs with Goat Cheese

Total time: 50 min

Prep time: 15 min

Cook time: 35 min

Yield: 8 servings

Ingredients:

- 1 tbsp. Of tallow
- 2 lbs. Of ground beef
- 1 organic egg
- 1 grated onion
- 1/2 cup of almond milk (unsweetened)
- 1 cup of red wine
- 1/2 bunch of chopped parsley
- 1/2 cup of almond flour
- Salt and ground pepper to taste
- 1/2 tbsp. Of dry oregano
- 4 oz. Of hard goat cheese cut into cubes

Directions:

1. Preheat oven to 400°f.

2. Grease a baking pan with tallow.

3. In a large bowl, combine all ingredients except goat cheese.

4. Knead the mixture until ingredients: are evenly combined.

5. Make small meatballs and place them in a prepared baking dish.

6. Place one cube of cheese on each meatball.

7. Bake for 30 - 35 minutes.

8. Serve hot.

18.Parisian Schnitzel

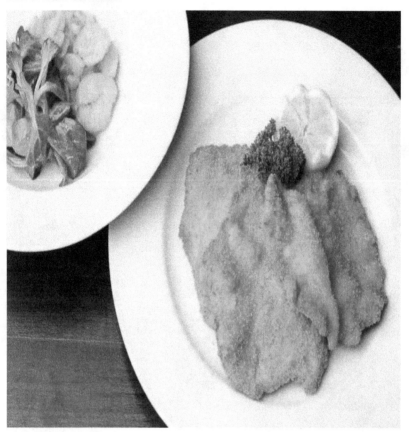

Total time: 25 min

Prep time: 15 min

Cook time: 10 min

Yield: 4 servings

Ingredients:

- Four veal steaks; thin schnitzel
- Salt and ground black pepper
- 2 tbsp. Of butter
- Three eggs from free-range chickens

- 4 tbsp. Of almond flour

Directions:

1. With salt and pepper, season the steaks.

2. Heat butter over medium heat in a large nonstick frying pan.

3. Beat the eggs in a bowl.

4. In a bowl, add the almond flour.

5. Using almond flour to roll each steak, then add and dip in the beaten eggs.

6. Fry each side for around 3 minutes.

7. Serve instantly.

19.Kato Beef Stroganoff

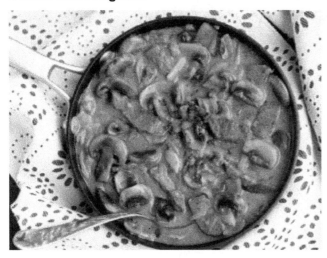

Prep time: 5 minutes

Cook time: 30 minutes

Yield: 6 servings

Ingredients:

- 2 lbs. Of rump or round steak or stewing steak

- 4 tbsp. Of olive oil

- 2 green onions, finely chopped

- 1 grated tomato
- 2 tbsp. Ketchup (without sugar)
- 1 cup of button mushrooms
- 1/2 cup of bone broth
- 1 cup of sour cream
- Salt and black pepper to taste

Directions:

1. Break the beef into strips and sauté it in a large pan for frying.
2. Add the chopped onion and a pinch of salt and roast at a medium temperature for around 20 minutes.
3. Add the ketchup and mushrooms and mix for 3 - 5 minutes.
4. Pour the sour cream and bone broth and simmer for 3 to 4 minutes.
5. Remove and taste from the fire and change the salt and pepper to taste.
6. Serve it warm.

20.Meatloaf with Gruyere

Total time: 55 min

Prep time: 15 min

Cook time: 40 min

Yields: 6 servings

Ingredients:

- 1 1/2 lbs. Ground beef
- 1 cup ground almonds
- 1 large egg from free-range chickens
- 1/2 cup grated gruyere cheese
- 1 tsp. Fresh parsley finely chopped
- 1 scallion finely chopped
- 1/2 tsp. Ground cumin

- 3 eggs boiled
- 2 tbsp. Of fresh grass-fed butter, melted

Directions:

1. Preheat the oven to 350 degrees F.

2. Combine all the ingredients in a large bowl (except for the eggs and butter).

3. Use your hands to combine the mixture properly.

4. Shape the mixture into a roll and put the sliced hard-boiled eggs in the middle.

5. To a 5x9 inch loaf pan greased with melted butter, switch the meatloaf.

6. Put in the oven and cook for 40 minutes, or until the temperature inside is 160 °F.

7. Take it out of the oven and let it sit for 10 minutes.

8. Slicing and cooking.

9.

21.Roasted Filet Mignon in Foil

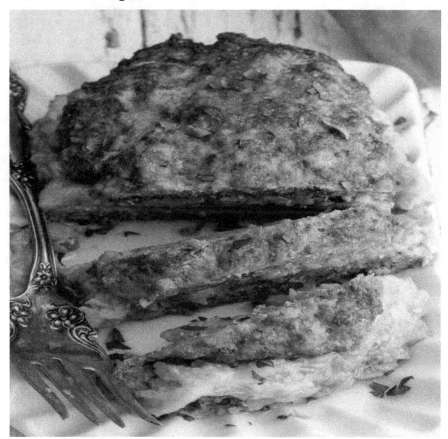

Total time: 60 min

Prep time: 15 min

Cook time: 45 min

Yield: 8 servings

Ingredients:

- 3 lbs. Filet mignon in one piece
- Salt to taste and ground black pepper
- 1 tsp. Of garlic powder
- 1 tsp. Of onion powder

- 1 tsp. Of cumin
- 4 tbsp. Of olive oil

Directions:

1. Preheat the oven to 425°f.

2. Rinse and clean the filet mignon, removing all fats, or ask your butcher to do it for you.

3. Season with salt and pepper, garlic powder, onion powder and cumin.

4. Wrap filet mignon in foil and place in a roasting pan, drizzle with the olive oil.

5. Roast for 15 minutes per pound for medium-rare or to desired doneness.

6. Remove from the oven and allow to rest for 10 -15 minutes before serving.

22.Stewed Beef with Green Beans

Prep time: 10 minutes

Cook time: 50 minutes

Yield: 8 servings

Ingredients:

- 1/2 cup olive oil
- 1 1/2 lbs. Beef cut into cubes
- 2 scallions, finely chopped
- 2 cups water
- 1 lb. Fresh green beans - trimmed and cut diagonally in half
- 1 bay leaf
- 1 grated tomato
- 1/2 cup fresh mint leaves, finely chopped
- 1 tsp. Fresh or dry rosemary
- Salt and freshly ground pepper to taste

Directions:

1. Chop the beef into cubes that are 1 inch thick.

2. In a big pot, heat olive oil over high heat. Sauté the beef and sprinkle it with a pinch of salt and pepper for around 4 - 5 minutes.

3. Add the scallions and mix and sauté until softened for around 3 - 4 more minutes. For 2-3 minutes, pour water and cook.

4. Add the grated tomato and bay leaf. Cook for 5 minutes or so; reduce the heat to medium-low. For about 15 minutes, cover and boil.

5. Add the rosemary, green beans, salt, fresh ground pepper and ample water to cover all the ingredients. Simmer softly, until the green beans are tender, for 15 - 20 minutes.

6. Sprinkle with the rosemary and mint, carefully blend and extract from the sun. Serve it warm.

23.Garlic Herb Butter Roasted Radishes

Total time: 20 min

Prep time: 10 min

Cook time: 10 min

Yield: (4per servings)

Ingredients:

- 1-pound of radishes
- 2 tablespoons of unsalted butter, melted
- 1/2 teaspoon of garlic powder
- ½ teaspoon of dried parsley
- 1/4 teaspoon of dried oregano
- 1/4 teaspoon of ground black pepper

Directions:

1. Separate the roots from the radishes and cut them into parts.

2. Then, in a small bowl, spread butter and seasonings. Swirl the radishes in the herbal butter and place them in the Air Fryer basket.

3. Fix the temperature for 10 minutes to 350° F and adjust the timer.

4. Throw the radishes halfway through the cooking cycle in the Air Fryer basket. Enable it to cool until the edges begin to turn orange.

5. Serve it hot and drink it!

24.Sausage-Stuffed Mushroom Caps

Total time: 20 min

Prep time: 10 min

Cook time: 10 min

Yield: (4per servings)

Ingredients:

- 6 large portobello mushroom caps
- ½-pound of Italian sausage
- 1/4 cup of chopped onion
- 2 tablespoons of blanched finely ground almond flour
- ¼ cup of grated Parmesan cheese
- 1 teaspoon of minced fresh garlic

Directions:

1. To hollow each cap of the mushrooms, use a spoon and save the scraps.

2. Brown the sausage for approximately 10 minutes in a medium saucepan over medium pressure,

3. Or until completely cooked and there is no residual pink. Drain the mushroom, cabbage, almond flour, parmesan, and garlic and then add preserved scrapings. Gently fold the ingredients together and proceed to cook for another minute, then extract them from the flames.

4. Scoop the mixture equally into mushroom caps and put the caps in a bowl of 6 rounds. Place the pan in an Air Fryer basket.

5. Set the temperature to 375° F and set the eight-minute timer.

6. When frying is finished, the tops will be browned and bubbled, and serve gently.

25.Cheesy Cauliflower Tots

Total time: 20 min

Prep time: 10 min

Cook time: 10 min

Yield: (4per servings)

Ingredients:

- 1 large head of cauliflower
- 1 cup of shredded mozzarella cheese
- 1/2 cup of grated Parmesan cheese
- 1large egg
- 1/4 teaspoon of garlic powder
- 1/4 teaspoon of dried parsley
- 1/8 teaspoon of onion powder

Directions:

1. On the stovetop, fill a huge pot with 2 cups of water and place a steamer in the oven. Get the bath to a boil. Break the cauliflower into a flower and put the pot and lid on a steamer box.

2. Let the cauliflower steam for 7 minutes, until tender. Place the steamer basket in your cheesecloth or clean kitchen towel and let it cool. To remove as much excess humidity as possible, push on the sink. The mixture would be too fragile to form into tots if not all of the moisture is extracted. Mash down with a razor into a smooth consistency.

3. Place the cauliflower and add the mozzarella, parmesan, cheese, garlic powder, parsley, and onion powder in a large mixing cup. Remove before you mix properly. Smooth but easy to mold, the mix should be.

4. Roll the mixture into a tot shape by taking 2 teaspoons of the mixture. Repeat for the remaining mixture. In the Air Fryer, bring the basket in.

5. Fix the temperature for 12 minutes to 320° F and set the timer.

6. Switch the tots halfway through the cooking time. Cauliflower tots, when fully baked, should be golden. Serve it hot.

26.Crispy Brussels sprouts

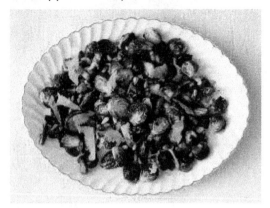

Total time: 20 min

Prep time: 10 min

Cook time: 10 min

Yield: (4per servings)

Ingredients:

- 1-pound of Brussels sprouts
- 1 tablespoon of coconut oil
- 1 tablespoon of unsalted butter, melted

Directions:

1. Every sprout of loose leaves from Brussels is removed and cut in half.
2. Spray it with coconut oil and drop it in the Air Fryer basket.
3. Set the temperature to 400 degrees F and for 10 minutes, change the timer. Depending on how they start browning, you might want to stir gently halfway through the cooking process.
4. When fully baked, they should be tender with darker caramelized spots. Drizzle with the molten butter and cut it out of the bowl of the fryer. Serve without hesitation.

27.Zucchini Parmesan Chips

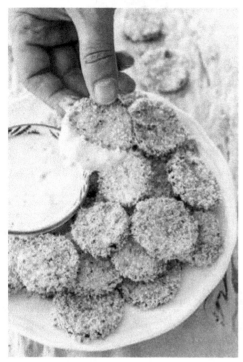

Total time: 20 min

Prep time: 10 min

Cook time: 10 min

Yield: 1 serving

Ingredients:

- 2 medium zucchinis
- 1-ounce of pork rinds
- 1/2 cup of grated Parmesan cheese
- 1 large egg

Directions:

1. 1/4-inch thick slices of a zucchini slice. To extract the excess moisture, place 30 minutes between two layers of paper towels or a clean kitchen towel.

2. In a food processor, put pork rinds and pulse until finely ground. Pour into a medium bowl and blend with parmesan.

3. In a small saucepan, pound the potato.

4. In the egg mixture, dip the zucchini slices and then cover as deeply as possible in the pork rind mixture. Put each slice carefully in a single layer of the Air Fryer bowl, working in batches as needed.

5. Adjust the temperature and set a 10-minute timer to 320° F.

6. Halfway into cooking time, flip chips. Serve hot and enjoy!

28.Roasted Garlic

Total time: 20 min

Prep time: 10 min

Cook time: 10 min

Yield: 1 serving

Ingredients:

- 1 medium head of garlic
- 2 teaspoons of avocado oil

Directions:

1. Strip any excess peel hanging from the garlic still cover the cloves. Shutdown

1/4 of the garlic handle, with clove tips visible.

2. Avocado oil spray. Place the garlic head in a small sheet of aluminum foil, and enclose it completely. Place it in the basket for Air Fryer.

3. Set the temperature to 400° F and change the timer for 20 minutes. If your garlic head is a little smaller, take 15 minutes to check it out.

4. Ail should be golden brown and very fluffy when finished.

5. Cloves should pop out to eat and be scattered or sliced quickly. In the refrigerator, lock in an airtight jar for up to 5 days. You can also freeze individual cloves on a baking sheet, then lock them together until frozen in a freezer-safe storage jar.

29.Kale Chips

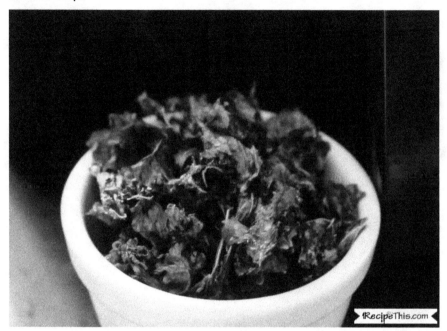

Total time: 20 min

Prep time: 10 min

Cook time: 10 min

Yield: 2 servings

Ingredients:

- 4 cups of steamed kale
- 2 teaspoons of avocado oil
- 1/2 teaspoon of salt

Directions:

1. Sprinkle the kale in a big bowl of avocado oil and sprinkle it with ice. Place it inside the Air Fryer basket.

2. Adjust the temperature and set a 5-minute timer to 400° f.

3. The kale will be crispy until it was done. Serve without hesitation.

30.Buffalo Cauliflower

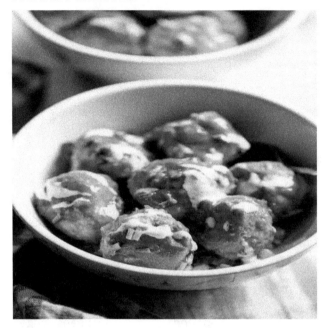

Total time: 20 min

Prep time: 10 min

Cook time: 10 min

Yield: 4 servings

Ingredients:

- 4 cups of cauliflower florets
- 2 tablespoons of salted butter, melted
- 1/2 (1-ounce)dry ranch seasoning packet
- 1/4 cup of buffalo sauce

Directions:

1. Toss the cauliflower with the butter and dry the ranch in a wide bowl. Place the basket in the Air Fryer.

2. Change the temperature and set the timer to 400°F for 5 minutes.

3. Shake the basket during the cooking process two to three times. Remove the coli flower from the fryer basket when tender and toss in the buffalo sauce. Serve it hot.

31.Green Bean Casserole

Total time: 20 min

Prep time: 10 min

Cook time: 10 min

Yield: 4 servings

Ingredients:

- 4 tablespoons of unsalted butter
- 1/4 cup of diced yellow onion
- 1/2 cup of chopped white mushrooms
- 1/2 cup of heavy whipping cream
- 1 ounce of full-Fat: cream cheese
- 1/2 cup of chicken broth
- 1/4 teaspoon of xanthan gum 1-pound fresh green beans, edges trimmed
- ½ ounce of pork rinds, finely ground

Directions:

1. Melt butter over low heat in a medium saucepan. Before they become soft and fragrant, cook the onion and mushrooms for around 3–5 minutes.

2. Add the hard whipped cream, cream cheese, and broth to the saucepan. Before, whisk quickly. Bring it to a boil, then drop it to a simmer. Sprinkle the gum with xanthan gum in the pan and fry.

3. Break the green beans into 2 parts and arrange them in a round 4-cup baking dish. Spillover those with the sauce mixture and stir until fried. With the rinds of the ground pork, fill the dish.

4. Fix the temperature to 320 degrees F and for 15 minutes, set the timer.

5. Top fork-tender when fully fried, golden and green beans. Soft serving.

32.Cilantro Lime Roasted Cauliflower

Total time: 20 min

Prep time: 10 min

Cook time: 10 min

Yield: 4 servings

Ingredients:

- 2 cups of chopped cauliflower florets
- 2 tablespoons of coconut oil, melted
- 2teaspoons of chili powder
- 1/2 teaspoon of garlic powder
- 1 medium lime
- 2 tablespoons of chopped cilantro

Directions:

1. In a big bowl of coconut oil, combine the cauliflower. Using ground chili and garlic to scatter. Put some seasoned cauliflower in the Air Fryer basket.

2. Set the temperature to 350 degrees F and change the seven-minute timer. The cauliflower gets wet on the sides and starts to turn golden. Set it down in a bowl to eat.

3. Break the lime into quarters and spill over it with cauliflower milk. Coriander garnish.

33.Dinner Rolls

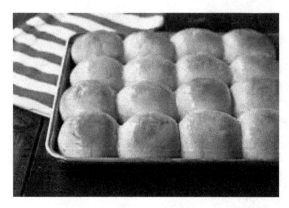

Total time: 20 min

Prep time: 10 min

Cook time: 10 min

Yield: 4 servings

Ingredients:

- 1 cup of shredded mozzarella cheese
- 1 ounce of full-Fat: cream cheese
- 1 cup of blanched finely ground almond flour
- 1/4 cup of ground flaxseed
- ½ teaspoon of baking powder
- 1 large egg

Directions:

1. Place the mozzarella, cream cheese, and almond flour in a large microwave-safe oven. Until flat, blend.

2. Substitute until smooth and thoroughly mixed with flaxseed, baking powder, and egg. Pulse for another 15 seconds if it gets too stiff.

3. Separate the dough into six pieces and roll the dough into balls. Put the Air Fryer balls in the basket.

4. Turn to 320° F and set the 12-minute timer.

5. Enable the rolls to cool completely before eating.

34.Fiery Stuffed Peppers

Preparation time: 20 minutes

Cooking time: 20 minutes

Servings: 4

Ingredients:

- 4 medium green peppers, seeds and stems removed
- 150 g lean minced meat
- 80g grated cheddar cheese, divided
- ½ cup tomato sauce, divided
- ½ tsp. Dried mango powder
- ½ tsp. Chili powder
- ½ tsp. Turmeric powder
- 1 tsp. Worcestershire sauce
- 1 tsp. Coriander powder
- 1 onion, minced
- 1 clove garlic, minced
- 2 tsp., minced coriander leaves
- 1 tsp. Vegetable oil

Directions:

1. Start by setting the oven to 390 degrees f for your air fryer toast.

2. Cook the peppers in salted boiling water for 3 minutes, then move them to a dish.

3. Apply the oil over medium-low heat to a small saucepan and sauté the onion and garlic for 1-2 minutes, then remove from the heat.

4. Combine all the ingredients, except half the cheese and tomato sauce, in a big bowl.

5. With the beef mixture, stuff the peppers and cover with the remaining cheese and tomato sauce.

6. Lightly oil the basket and place the 4 stuffed peppers from your air fryer toast oven.

7. Cook for 15 to 20 minutes or before you want it cooked. Enjoy!

35.Beef and veggies stir fry

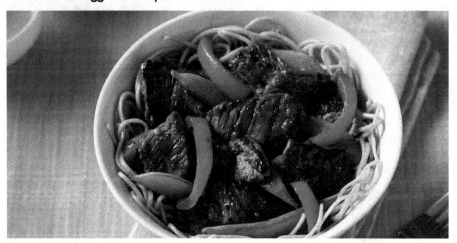

Preparation time: 45 minutes

Cooking time: 15 minutes

Servings: 4

Ingredients:

- 450g beef sirloin, cut into strips

- 1 yellow pepper, sliced

- 1 red pepper, sliced

- 1 green pepper, sliced

- 1 broccoli, cut into florets

- 1 large red onion, sliced

- 1 large white onion, sliced

- 1 tsp. Sesame oil

- For the marinade:
- 2 tsp. Minced garlic
- 1 tbsp. Low sodium soy sauce
- ¼ cup hoisin sauce
- ¼ cup water
- 1 tsp. Sesame oil
- 1 tsp. Ground ginger

Directions:

1. In a wide bowl, begin by whisking all the marinade ingredients. Add in the strips of beef and toss well, so all the bits are covered equally. Using cling wrap to protect it and let it stay for 30 minutes in the fridge.

2. Combine all the vegetables and the sesame oil and place the toast oven in the basket of your air fryer at 200 degrees F. For 5 minutes, cook.

3. Move the vegetables to a bowl and put the meat in your toast oven's air fryer basket.

4. Be sure that the marinade is drained. Increase the temperature and simmer for 5 minutes, to 360 degrees f. Shake the meat and cook for an additional 3 minutes, or until needed.

5. Attach the vegetables and simmer for an extra 2 minutes.

6. Serve on a steamed rice bed. Enjoy!

36.Air Fried Chili Beef with Toasted Cashews

Preparation time: 10 minutes

Cooking time: 25 minutes

Servings: 24

Ingredients:

- ½ tablespoon extra-virgin olive oil or canola oil
- 450g sliced lean beef
- 2 teaspoons red curry paste
- 1 teaspoon liquid stevia, optional

- 2 tablespoons fresh lime juice
- 2 teaspoon fish sauce
- 1 cup green capsicum, diced
- ½ cup water
- 24 toasted cashews
- 1 teaspoon arrowroot starch

Directions:

1. Set the oven to 375 degrees f for your air fryer toast.
2. Mix the beef and olive oil and fry for about 15 minutes until the inside is no longer yellow, rotating twice.
3. Apply the red curry paste and simmer for a few more minutes.
4. Mix the stevia, lime juice, fish sauce, capsicum and water in a big pot; boil for about 10 minutes.
5. To make a paste, mix cooked arrowroot with water; stir the paste into the sauce to thicken it.
6. Attach the fried cashews and remove the pan from the sun. Serve.

37.Beef Stir Fry W/ Red Onions & Peppers

Preparation time: 10 minutes

Cooking time: 10 minutes

Servings: 4

Ingredients:

- 450g grass-fed flank steak, thinly sliced strips
- 1 tablespoon rice wine
- 2 teaspoons balsamic vinegar
- Pinch of sea salt
- Pinch of pepper
- 3 teaspoons extra-virgin olive oil

- 1 large yellow onion, thinly chopped

- 1/2 red bell pepper, thinly sliced

- 1/2 green bell pepper, thinly sliced

- 1 tablespoon toasted sesame seeds

- 1 teaspoon crushed red pepper flakes

Directions:

Place meat in a bowl; stir in rice wine and vinegar, sea salt and pepper. Toss to coat well.

Set your air fryer toast oven to 375 degrees f.

Add the meat and olive and cook for about 3-5 minutes or until the meat is browned.

Heat the remaining oil on a stovetop pan and sauté onions for about 2 minutes or until caramelized; stir in pepper and cook for 2 minutes more.

Add the caramelized onions to the air fryer toast oven and stir in sesame seeds and red pepper flakes and cook for 1-2 minutes. Serve hot!

38.Air Fryer Toast Oven Italian Beef

Preparation time: 10 minutes

Cooking time: 1 hour 30 minutes

Servings: 8

Ingredients:

- 1200g grass-fed chuck roast

- 6 cloves garlic

- 1 tsp. Marjoram

- 1 tsp. Basil

- 1 tsp. Oregano

- 1/2 tsp. Ground ginger

- 1 tsp. Onion powder

- 2 tsp. Garlic powder

- 1 tsp. Salt

- 1/4 cup apple cider vinegar
- 1 cup beef broth

Directions:

1. Cut slits in the roast with a sharp knife and then stuff with garlic cloves. In a bowl, whisk together marjoram, basil, oregano, ground ginger, onion powder, garlic powder, and salt until well blended; rub the seasoning all over the roast and place in a large air fryer toast oven pan.

2. Add vinegar and broth and lock lid; cook at 400 degrees f for 90 minutes. Take the roast out and then shred meat with a fork. Serve along with cooking juices.

39.Healthy Quinoa Bowl with Grilled Steak & Veggies

Preparation time: 10 minutes

Cooking time: 20 minutes

Servings: 4

Ingredients:

- 2 cups quinoa
- 16 ounces steak, cut into bite-size pieces
- 1 cup baby arugula
- 1 cup sweet potato slices
- 1 cup red pepper, chopped
- 1 cup scallions, chopped
- 1/2 cup toasted salted pepitas
- 2 tsp. Fresh cilantro leaves
- 2 cups microgreens
- 2 tbsp. Tomato sauce
- 2 tbsp. Extra-virgin olive oil
- Kosher salt
- Black pepper
- 1 tbsp. Fresh lime juice

Directions:

1. In your instant cooker, cook quinoa as needed.

2. Meanwhile, in your air-fryer toast oven, grill steak to medium rare for around 15 minutes at 350 degrees f. Grill the scallions, red pepper and sweet potatoes until tender, along with the beef.

3. Top with grilled beef, scallions, veggies, pepitas, cilantro, and microgreens. Place cooked quinoa in a bowl.

4. Combine the oil, tomato sauce, salt, and pepper in a small bowl until well blended; drizzle over the steak mixture and serve with lime juice.

27. Pork and Mixed Greens Salad

Preparation time: 10 minutes

Cooking time: 15 minutes

Servings: 4

Ingredients:

- 2 pounds pork tenderloin, slice into 1-inch slices
- 1 teaspoon dried marjoram
- 6 cups mixed salad greens
- 1 (8-ounce) package button mushrooms, sliced
- 1/3 cup low-sodium low-fat vinaigrette dressing

Directions:

1. Combine the olive oil and the pork slices. Toss it to coat it.

2. Sprinkle the marjoram and pepper with them and rub them onto the pork.

3. Grill the pork in batches in an air fryer until the pork on a meat thermometer hits at least 145 °f.

4. Combine the red bell pepper, salad greens, and mushrooms. Gently toss.

5. Add the slices to the salad until cooked.

6. Drizzle and toss softly with the vinaigrette. Immediately serve.

40.Pork Satay

Preparation time: 15 minutes

Cooking time: 14 minutes

Servings: 4

Ingredients:

- 1 (1-pound) pork tenderloin, cut into 1½-inch cubes
- ¼ cup minced onion
- 2 garlic cloves, minced
- 2 tablespoons freshly squeezed lime juice, coconut milk, curry powder
- 2 tablespoons unsalted peanut butter

Directions:

1. Combine the ham, ginger, garlic, jalapeño, coconut milk, lime juice, peanut butter, and curry powder with the mixture. Place it aside at room temperature for 10 minutes.
2. From the marinade, take the pork out. Marinade Reserve.
3. Onto approximately 8 bamboo skewers, string the pork. With the reserved marinade, grill and clean once, before the pork on a meat thermometer hits at least 145 °f. Discard every marinade that exists. Immediately serve.

41.Pork Burgers with Red Cabbage Salad

Preparation time: 20 minutes

Cooking time: 9 minutes

Servings: 4

Ingredients:

- ½ cup greek yogurt
- 2 tablespoons low-sodium mustard, paprika
- 1 tablespoon lemon juice
- ¼ cup red cabbage, carrots
- 1-pound lean ground pork

Directions:

1. Combine 1 tablespoon of mustard, lemon juice, cabbage, and carrots with the yogurt; blend and cool.

2. Combine the bacon, 1 tablespoon of mustard left, and the paprika. Mold into eight little patties.

3. Insert the sliders into the basket of the air fryer. Grill with a meat thermometer until the sliders register 165 ° f as checked.

4. By putting some of the lettuce greens on a bun bottom, arrange the burgers. Cover it with a slice of onion, tacos, and a combination of cabbage. Attach the top of the bun and quickly serve.

42.Crispy Mustard Pork Tenderloin

Preparation time: 10 minutes

Cooking time: 12 to 16 minutes

Servings: 4

Ingredients:

- 3 tablespoons low-sodium grainy mustard
- ¼ teaspoon dry mustard powder
- 1 (1-pound) pork tenderloin
- ¼ cup ground walnuts
- 2 tablespoons cornstarch

Directions:

9. Stir together the mustard, olive oil, and mustard powder. Spread this mixture over the pork.

10. On a plate, mix the bread crumbs, walnuts, and cornstarch. Dip the mustard-coated pork into the crumb mixture to coat.

11. Air-fry the pork until it registers at least 145°f on a meat thermometer. Slice to serve.

43.Apple Pork Tenderloin

Preparation time: 10 minutes

Cooking time: 14 to 19 minutes

Servings: 4

Ingredients:

- 1 (1-pound) pork tenderloin, cut into 4 pieces
- 1 tablespoon apple butter
- 2 granny smith apples or Jonagold apples, sliced
- ½ teaspoon dried marjoram
- 1/3 cup apple juice

Directions:

1. Rub the apple butter and olive oil with each slice of pork.
2. Mix together the bacon, apples, 3 celery, 1 marjoram, 1 cabbage, and apple juice.
3. Place the bowl in the fryer and roast until the pork on a meat thermometer hits at least 145 ° f, and the apples and vegetables are tender. During cooking, stir once. Immediately serve.

44.Espresso-Grilled Pork Tenderloin

Preparation time: 15 minutes

Cooking time: 9 to 11 minutes

Servings: 4

Ingredients:

- 2 teaspoons espresso powder
- 1 teaspoon ground paprika
- ½ teaspoon dried marjoram
- 1 tablespoon honey, lemon juice, brown sugar
- 1 (1-pound) pork tenderloin

Directions:

Combine the brown sugar, marjoram, paprika, and espresso powder.

Stir in the olive oil, lemon juice and honey until well combined.

Spread the honey mixture over the pork and let it rest at room temperature for 10 minutes.

In the air fryer basket, roast the tenderloin until the pork reports at least 145°f on a meat thermometer. To cook, slice the beef.

45.Garlic Lamb Chops with Thyme

Preparation time: 10 minutes

Cooking time: 30 minutes

Servings: 4

Ingredients:

- 4 lamb chops
- 1 garlic clove, peeled
- 1 tbsp. plus
- 2 tsp. olive oil
- ½ tbsp. oregano
- ½ tbsp. thyme
- ⅓ tsp. salt
- ¼ tsp. black pepper

Directions:

1. Preheat the fryer to 390 f for air. Coat the clove of garlic with 1 tsp. Olive oil and put for 10 minutes in the air fryer. Meanwhile, with the remaining olive oil, combine the herbs and seasonings.

2. Squeeze the hot roasted garlic clove into the herb mixture using a towel or a mitten, and stir to blend. Coat the mixture well with the lamb chops, and put them in the air fryer. For 8 to 12 minutes, cook.

3.

46.Lamb Meatloaf

Preparation time: 15 minutes

Cooking time: 40 minutes

Servings: 4

Ingredients:

- 2 lb. Lamb, ground
- 4 scallions; chopped
- 1 egg
- A drizzle of olive oil
- 2 tbsp. Tomato sauce
- 2 tbsp. Parsley; chopped
- 2 tbsp. Cilantro; chopped
- ¼ tsp. Cinnamon powder
- 1 tsp. Coriander, ground
- 1 tsp. Lemon juice
- ½ tsp. Hot paprika
- 1 tsp. Cumin, ground
- A pinch of salt and black pepper

Directions:

1. Combine the lamb in a bowl with the rest of the ingredients, except for the oil, and mix very well.

2. Grease a loaf pan that suits the oil in the air fryer, add the lamb mix and mold the meatloaf

3. Place the pan in an air fryer and cook for 35 minutes at 380 °f. Slicing and serving

4.

47.Lamb Chops and Mint Sauce

Preparation time: 10 minutes

Cooking time: 29 minutes

Servings: 4

Ingredients:

- 8 lamb chops
- 1 cup mint; chopped
- 1 garlic clove; minced
- 2 tbsp. Olive oil
- Juice of 1 lemon
- A pinch of salt and black pepper

Directions:

1. Combine all the ingredients in a blender, except the lamb, and pulse well.

2. Rub lamb chops with the mint sauce, place them in your air fryer's basket and cook at 400°f for 12 minutes on each side

3. Divide and serve everything between plates.

4.

48.Rosemary Roasted Lamb Cutlets

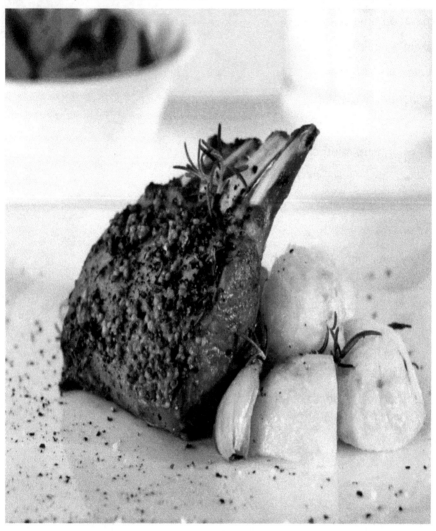

Preparation time: 15 minutes

Cooking time: 35 minutes

Servings: 4

Ingredients:

- 8 lamb cutlets

- 2 garlic cloves; minced
- 2 tbsp. Rosemary; chopped
- 2 tbsp. Olive oil
- A pinch of salt and black pepper
- A pinch of cayenne pepper

Directions:

1. Take a bowl and mix the rest of the ingredients with the lamb: rub well.
2. Place the lamb in the fryer's basket and cook for 30 minutes at 380°f, flipping halfway. Divide between plates and serve the cutlets

49.Seasoned Lamb

Preparation time: 15 minutes

Cooking time: 40 minutes

Servings: 4

Ingredients:

- 1 lb. Lamb leg; boneless and sliced
- ½ cup walnuts; chopped
- 2 garlic cloves; minced
- 1 tbsp. Parsley; chopped
- 1 tbsp. Rosemary; chopped
- 2 tbsp. Olive oil
- ¼ tsp. Red pepper flakes
- ½ tsp. Mustard seeds
- ½ tsp. Italian seasoning
- A pinch of salt and black pepper

Directions:

1. Take a bowl and combine the lamb with all the ingredients: rub well except the walnuts and parsley, place the slices in the basket of your air fryer and cook for 35 minutes at 370 ° F, flipping the meat halfway.

2. Spread the parsley and walnuts on top and serve with a side salad. Split between dishes.

50. Herbed Lamb

Preparation time: 15 minutes

Cooking time: 40 minutes

Servings: 4

Ingredients:

- 8 lamb cutlets
- ¼ cup mustard
- 2 garlic cloves; minced
- 1 tbsp. Oregano; chopped
- 1 tbsp. Mint chopped.
- 1 tbsp. Chives; chopped
- 1 tbsp. Basil; chopped
- A drizzle of olive oil
- A pinch of salt and black pepper

Directions:

1. Take a bowl and mix the rest of the ingredients with the lamb: rub well.
2. Place the cutlets in the basket of your air fryer and cook on each side at 380°f for 15 minutes.
3. Divide and serve with a side salad between dishes.

51. Rack of Lamb

Preparation time: 5 minutes

Cooking time: 10 minutes

Servings: 2 to 4

Ingredients:

- 1 rack of lamb
- 2 tbsp. Of dried rosemary

- 1 tbsp. Of dried thyme
- 2 tsp. Of minced garlic
- Salt
- Pepper
- 4 tbsp. Of olive oil

Directions:

1. Start by combining the herbs, mixing the rosemary, thyme, garlic, salt, pepper, and olive oil in a small bowl and combine well.

2. Rub the mixture all over the lamb, then. Place the lamb rack inside the air fryer. Set the temperature for about 10 minutes, to 360f.

3. After 10 minutes, use the method above to calculate the internal temperature of the lamb rack. It will be 145 f If you want an uncommon one.

4. That will be 160 f if you want a medium. If you'd like to do well, it would be 170 f. Remove the bowls, then serve.

52.Lamb Sirloin Steak

Preparation time: 40 minutes

Cooking time: 15 minutes

Servings: 2 to 4

Ingredients:

- ½ onions
- 4 slices of ginger
- 5 cloves of garlic
- 1 tsp. of garam masala
- 1 tsp. Of ground fennel
- 1 tsp. Of ground cinnamon
- ½ tsp. Of ground cardamom
- 1 tsp. Of cayenne
- 1 tsp. Of salt

- 1 lb. Of boneless lamb sirloin steaks

Directions:

1. Add all the ingredients to a blender bowl, except the lamb chops.

2. Pulse and blend until the onion and all ingredients are finely minced: blend for around 3 to 4 minutes.

3. Place the chops of the lamb into a side dish. To allow the marinade to penetrate better, use a knife to slice the meat and fat.

4. Toss well the mixed spice paste and combine well. Enable the mixture to rest for 30 minutes or in the refrigerator for up to 24 hours.

5. For about 15 minutes, allow your air fryer to 330 f and place the lamb steaks in the air fryer basket in a single layer and cook, flipping halfway through.

6. Ensure that the meat has reached an inner temperature of 150f for medium-well, using a meat thermometer, and serve.

53.Beef Pork Meatballs

Preparation time: 10 minutes

Cooking time: 20 minutes

Servings: 6

Ingredients:

- 1 lb. Ground beef
- 1 lb. Ground pork
- 1/2 cup Italian breadcrumbs
- 1/3 cup milk
- 1/4 cup onion, diced
- 1/2 teaspoon garlic powder
- 1 teaspoon Italian seasoning
- 1 egg
- 1/4 cup parsley chopped
- 1/4 cup shredded parmesan

- Salt and pepper to taste

Directions:

1. In a bowl, carefully mix the beef with all the other meatball ingredients.

2. Create tiny meatballs out of this combination, then put them in the basket of the air fryer.

3. Click the Air Fry Oven control button and switch the knob to pick the bake mode.

4. To set the cooking time to 20 minutes, click the time button and change the dial once again.

5. Now press the temp button to set the temperature at 400 degrees f and rotate the dial.

6. When preheated, put the basket of meatballs in the oven and close the lid.

7. When baked, turn the meatballs halfway through and then start cooking.

8. Serve it hot.

54.Beef Noodle Casserole

Preparation time: 10 minutes

Cooking time: 35 minutes

Servings: 6

Ingredients:

- 2 tablespoons olive oil
- 1 medium onion, chopped
- ½ lb. Ground beef
- 4 fresh mushrooms, sliced
- 1 cup pasta noodles, cooked
- 2 cups marinara sauce
- 1 teaspoon butter
- 4 teaspoons flour

- 1 cup milk
- 1 egg, beaten
- 1 cup cheddar cheese, grated

Directions:

12. Put a wok on moderate heat and add oil to heat.
13. Toss in onion and sauté until soft.
14. Stir in mushrooms and beef, then cook until meat is brown.
15. Add marinara sauce and cook it to a simmer.
16. Stir in pasta then spread this mixture in a casserole dish.
17. Prepare the sauce by melting butter in a saucepan over moderate heat.
18. Stir in flour and whisk well, pour in the milk.
19. Mix well and whisk ¼ cup sauce with egg, then return it to the saucepan.
20. Stir, cook for 1 minute, then pour this sauce over the beef.
21. Drizzle cheese over the beef casserole.
22. Press the "power button" of the air fry oven and turn the dial to select the "bake" mode.
23. Press the time button and again turn the dial to set the cooking time to 30 minutes.
24. Now push the temp button and rotate the dial to set the temperature at 350 degrees f.
25. Once preheated, place the casserole dish in the oven and close its lid.
26. Serve warm.

55.Saucy Beef Bake

Preparation time: 10 minutes

Cooking time: 36 minutes

Servings: 6

Ingredients:

- 2 tablespoons olive oil
- 1 large onion, diced

- 2 lbs. Ground beef
- 2 teaspoons salt
- 6 cloves garlic, chopped
- 1/2 cup red wine
- 6 cloves garlic, chopped
- 3 teaspoons ground cinnamon
- 2 teaspoons ground cumin
- 2 teaspoons dried oregano
- 1 teaspoon black pepper
- 1 can 28 oz. Crushed tomatoes
- 1 tablespoon tomato paste

Directions:

1. In a bowl, carefully mix the beef with all the other meatball ingredients.
2. Create tiny meatballs out of this combination, then put them in the basket of the air fryer.
3. Click the Air Fry Oven control button and switch the knob to pick the bake mode.
4. To set the cooking time to 20 minutes, click the time button and change the dial once again.
5. Now press the temp button to set the temperature at 400 degrees f and rotate the dial.
6. When preheated, put the basket of meatballs in the oven and close the lid.
7. When baked, turn the meatballs halfway through and then start cooking.
8. Serve it hot.

56.Beets and Arugula Salad

Total time: 20 min

Prep time: 10 min

Cook time: 10 min

Yield: 4 servings

Ingredients:

- 1 and ½ pounds of beets, peeled and quartered
- A drizzle of olive oil
- 2 teaspoons of orange zest, grated
- 2 tablespoons of cider vinegar
- ½ cup of orange juice
- 2 tablespoons of brown sugar
- 2 scallions, chopped
- 2 teaspoons of mustard
- 2 cups of arugula

Directions:

1. Rub the beets with the orange juice and oil, put them in your Air Fryer, and cook at 350 °F for 10 minutes.
2. Move the beet quarters to a bowl, add the scallions, arugula zest, and orange and blend.
3. In a separate dish, blend the sugar with the mustard and vinegar, blend properly, add the lettuce, whisk and eat.

57.Beet Tomato and Goat Cheese Mix

Total time: 45 min

Prep time: 20 min

Cook time: 25 min

Yield: 8 servings

Ingredients:

- 8 small beets, trimmed, peeled, and halved
- 1 red onion, sliced
- 4 ounces of goat cheese, crumbled
- 1 tablespoon of balsamic vinegar

- Salt and black pepper to the taste
- 2 tablespoons of sugar
- 1-pint mixed cherry tomatoes halved
- 2 ounces of pecans
- 2 tablespoons of olive oil

Directions:

1. Connect the beets to the Air Fryer, season with salt and pepper, cook for 14 minutes at 350 °F and move to a salad bowl.

2. Attach the carrot, pecans, and cherry tomatoes, and toss.

3. Mix the vinegar with the sugar and oil in another dish, stir well until the sugar dissolves, and add to the salad.

4. Add goat cheese as well, toss, and eat.

58.Broccoli Salad

Total time: 20 min

Prep time: 10 min

Cook time: 10 min

Yield: 8 servings

Ingredients:

- 1 broccoli head, florets separated
- 1 tablespoon of peanut oil
- 6 garlic cloves, minced
- 1 tablespoon of Chinese rice wine vinegar
- Salt and black pepper to the taste

Directions:

1. In a cup, mix broccoli with salt, pepper and half the oil, shake, switch to your Air Fryer, and cook at 350 °F for 8 minutes, shaking halfway through the fryer.

2. Transfer the broccoli and the leftover peanut oil, garlic and rice vinegar into a salad bowl, blend well and eat very nicely.

59.Brussels Sprouts and Tomatoes Mix

Total time: 15 min

Prep time: 5 min

Cook time: 10 min

Yield: 4 servings

Ingredients:

- 1-pound of Brussels sprouts, trimmed
- Salt and black pepper to the taste
- 6 cherry tomatoes, halved
- ¼ cup of green onions, chopped
- 1 tablespoon of olive oil

Directions:

1. Season Brussels with salt and pepper sprouts, put in your fryer and cook at 350 degrees F for 10 minutes.
2. Add salt, pepper, cherry tomatoes, olive oil, and green onions, blend well and eat. Put them in a cup.

60.Brussels Sprouts and Butter Sauce

Total time: 15 min

Prep time: 5 min

Cook time: 10 min

Yield: 4 servings

Ingredients:

- 1-pound of Brussels sprouts, trimmed
- Salt and black pepper to the taste
- ½ cup of bacon, cooked and chopped
- 1 tablespoon of mustard
- 1 tablespoon of butter
- 2 tablespoons dill, finely chopped

Directions:

1. In the Air Fryer, put the Brussels sprouts and cook them at 350 °F for 10 minutes.

2. Heat a skillet with the butter over medium-high heat, add the bacon, mustard, and dill and whisk well.

3. In Brussels, split the sprouts between bowls, drizzle the butter sauce all over, and eat.

61.Cheesy Brussels sprouts

Total time: 18 min

Prep time: 5 min

Cook time: 10 min

Yield: 4 servings

Ingredients:

- 1-pound of Brussels sprouts washed

- Juice of 1 lemon

- Salt and black pepper to the taste

- 2 tablespoons of butter

- 3 tablespoons of parmesan, grated

Directions:

1. Put the sprouts in the Brussels Air Fryer, cook them at 350 degrees F for 8 minutes, and position them on a tray.

2. Heat the butter in a skillet over medium heat, add the lemon juice, salt and pepper, stir well and add the Brussels sprouts.

3. Before the parmesan melts, add the parmesan, toss and serve.

62.Spicy Cabbage

Total time: 18 min

Prep time: 5 min

Cook time: 10 min

Yield: 4 servings

Ingredients:

- 1 cabbage, cut into 8 wedges
- 1 tablespoon of sesame seed oil
- 1 carrot, grated
- ¼ cup of apple cider vinegar
- ¼ cups of apple juice
- ½ teaspoon of cayenne pepper
- 1 teaspoon of red pepper flakes, crushed

Directions:

1. Combine cabbage with oil, carrot, vinegar, apple juice, cayenne, and pepper flakes, shake, put in preheated Air Fryer, and cook for 8 minutes at 350° F in a pan that suits your Air Fryer.

2. Divide and serve cabbage mixture on bowls.

63.Sweet Baby Carrots Dish

Total time: 20 min

Prep time: 5 min

Cook time: 15 min

Yield: 4 servings

Ingredients:

- 2 cups of baby carrots
- A pinch of salt and black pepper
- 1 tablespoon of brown sugar
- ½ tablespoon of butter, melted

Directions:

1. In a dish that fits your Air Fryer blend, add baby carrots with butter, salt, pepper and sugar, place in your Air Fryer, and cook at 350 °F for 10 minutes.

2. Divide and feed between bowls.

64.Collard Greens Mix

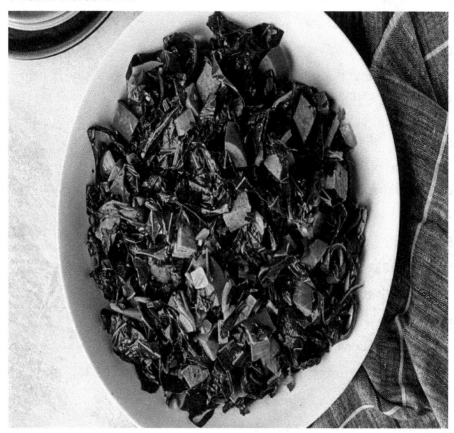

Total time: 20 min

Prep time: 5 min

Cook time: 15 min

Yield: 4 servings

Ingredients:

- 1 bunch of collard greens, trimmed
- 2 tablespoons of olive oil
- 2 tablespoons of tomato puree
- 1 yellow onion, chopped
- 3 garlic cloves, minced
- Salt and black pepper to the taste

- 1 tablespoon of balsamic vinegar
- 1 teaspoon of sugar

Directions:

1. In a bowl that matches your Air Fryer, mix the oil, garlic, vinegar, onion, and tomato puree and whisk.

2. Add the collard greens, salt, pepper and shake with the butter, stir in the Air Fryer and roast at 320 degrees F for 10 minutes.

3. Divide the collard greens into bowls and serve

65.Collard Greens and Turkey Wings

Total time: 30 min

Prep time: 10 min

Cook time: 25 min

Yield: 2 servings

Ingredients:

- 1 sweet onion, chopped
- 2 smoked turkey wings
- 2 tablespoons of olive oil
- 3 garlic cloves, minced
- 2 and ½ pounds of collard greens, chopped
- Salt and black pepper to the taste
- 2 tablespoons of apple cider vinegar
- 1 tablespoon of brown sugar
- ½ teaspoon of crushed red pepper

Directions:

1. Heat up a medium-hot saucepan that suits the grease of your Air Fryer, add the onions, stir and cook for 2 minutes.

2. Connect the garlic, the onions, the mustard, the salt, the pepper, the crushed red pepper, the cinnamon and the smoked turkey, add the preheated Air Fryer and cook at 350 degrees F for 15 minutes.

66.Herbed Eggplant and Zucchini Mix

Total time: 18 min

Prep time: 5 min

Cook time: 10 min

Yield: 4 servings

Ingredients:

- 1 eggplant, roughly cubed
- 3 zucchinis, roughly cubed
- 2 tablespoons of lemon juice
- Salt and black pepper to the taste
- 1 teaspoon of thyme, dried
- 1 teaspoon of oregano, dried
- 3 tablespoons of olive oil

Directions:

1. Place the eggplant in the bowl of the Air Fryer, add the zucchini, lemon juice, salt, pepper, thyme, oregano and olive oil, blend and place in the Air Fryer and cook for 8 minutes at 360 degrees F.

2. Divide into bowls and instantly serve.

67.Flavored Fennel

Total time: 18 min

Prep time: 5 min

Cook time: 10 min

Yield: 4 servings

Ingredients:

- 2 fennel bulbs, cut into quarters
- 3 tablespoons of olive oil
- Salt and black pepper to the taste
- 1 garlic clove, minced

- 1 red chili pepper, chopped
- ¾ cup of veggie stock
- Juice from ½ lemon
- ¼ cup of white wine
- ¼ cup of parmesan, grated

Directions:

1. Heat a medium-hot saucepan that fits the oil with your Air Fryer, add the garlic and chili pepper, stir and cook for 2 minutes.

2. Add the fennel, salt, pepper, stock, vinegar, lemon juice and parmesan, cover with a swirl, throw in the Air Fryer and cook at 350 °F for 6 minutes.

3. Divide them into plates.

68.Okra and Corn Salad

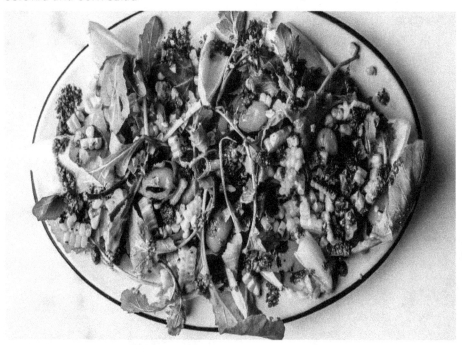

Total time: 20 min

Prep time: 5 min

Cook time: 15 min

Yield: 4 servings

Ingredients:

- 3 green bell peppers, chopped
- 2 tablespoons of olive oil
- 1 teaspoon of sugar
- 1-pound of okra, trimmed
- 6 scallions, chopped
- Salt and black pepper to the taste
- 28 ounces of canned tomatoes, chopped
- 1 cup of corn

Directions:

1. Heat a pan over medium-high heat that suits the oil with your Air Fryer, add bell peppers and scallions, blend and cook for 5 minutes.
2. Connect the okra, salt, pepper, sugar, tomatoes, and maize, stir, put in the Air Fryer and cook at 360 degrees F for 7 minutes.
3. Break the mixture of okra into plates and serve until wet.

69.Air Fried Leeks

Total time: 18 min

Prep time: 5 min

Cook time: 10 min

Yield: 4 servings

Ingredients:

- 4 leeks, washed, ends cut off and halved
- Salt and black pepper to the taste
- 1 tablespoon of butter, melted
- 1 tablespoon of lemon juice

Directions:

1. Rub the leeks with the melted butter, season with salt and pepper, add to the Air Fryer and cook at 350 degrees F for 7 minutes.

2. Set the lemon juice on a pan, drizzle it all over and eat.

70.Crispy Potatoes and Parsley

Total time: 20 min

Prep time: 5 min

Cook time: 15 min

Yield: 4 servings

Ingredients:

- 1-pound of gold potatoes, cut into wedges
- Salt and black pepper to the taste
- 2 tablespoons of olive
- Juice from ½ lemon
- ¼ cup of parsley leaves, chopped

Directions:

1. Rub the potatoes with salt, pepper, lemon juice and olive oil, add them to the Air Fryer and cook at 350 degrees F for 10 minutes.

2. Sprinkle on top of the parsley, break into bowls and eat.

71.Indian Turnips Salad

Total time: 22 min

Prep time: 7 min

Cook time: 15 min

Yield: 4 servings

Ingredients:

- 20 ounces of turnips, peeled and chopped
- 1 teaspoon of garlic, minced
- 1 teaspoon of ginger, grated
- 2 yellow onions, chopped

- 2 tomatoes, chopped
- 1 teaspoon of cumin, ground
- 1 teaspoon of coriander, ground
- 2 green chilies, chopped
- ½ teaspoon of turmeric powder
- 2 tablespoons of butter
- Salt and black pepper to the taste
- A handful of coriander leaves, chopped

Directions:

1. In a saucepan that fits your Air Fryer, heats the butter, melt it, add the green chilies, garlic, and ginger, stir and cook for 1 minute.

2. Add the onions, salt, pepper, tomatoes, turmeric, cumin, cilantro and turnips, stir, put in the Air Fryer and cook at 350 degrees F. for 10 minutes.

3. Break into cups, sprinkle with fresh coriander on top and serve.

72.Simple Stuffed Tomatoes

Total time: 25 min

Prep time: 10 min

Cook time: 15 min

Yield: 6 servings

Ingredients:

- 4 tomatoes, tops cut off and pulp scooped and chopped
- Salt and black pepper to the taste
- 1 yellow onion, chopped
- 1 tablespoon of butter
- 2 tablespoons of celery, chopped
- ½ cup of mushrooms, chopped
- 1 tablespoon of bread crumbs
- 1 cup of cottage cheese

- ¼ teaspoon of caraway seeds
- 1 tablespoon of parsley, chopped

Directions:

1. Heat a saucepan with the butter over medium heat, melt, add the onion and celery, stir and simmer for 3 minutes.

2. Link the mushrooms and tomato pulp and then stir and boil for 1 minute.

3. Add salt, pepper, crumbled bread, cheese, parsley, caraway seeds, stir, cook for another 4 minutes, and heat up.

4. With this blend, stuff the tomatoes, place them in the Air Fryer, and cook at 350 °F for 8 minutes.

5. Divide the stewed tomatoes into bowls and serve.

73.Indian Potatoes

Total time: 22 min

Prep time: 7 min

Cook time: 15 min

Yield: 4 servings

Ingredients:

- 1 tablespoon of coriander seeds
- 1 tablespoon of cumin seeds
- Salt and black pepper to the taste
- ½ teaspoon of turmeric powder
- ½ teaspoon of red chili powder
- 1 teaspoon of pomegranate powder
- 1 tablespoon of pickled mango, chopped
- 2 teaspoons of fenugreek, dried
- 5 potatoes, boiled, peeled, and cubed
- 2 tablespoons of olive oil

Directions:

1. Over medium pressure, heat a saucepan that suits the oil of your Air Fryer, add the coriander and cumin seeds, stir and simmer for 2 minutes.

2. Add cinnamon, pepper, turmeric, chili powder, mango, fenugreek, pomegranate powder and potatoes, blend, add Air Fryer and simmer at 360 °F for 10 minutes.

3. Divide and serve sweetly between bowls.

74.Broccoli and Tomatoes Air Fried Stew

Total time: 30 min

Prep time: 10 min

Cook time: 25 min

Yield: 2 servings

Ingredients:

- 1 broccoli head, florets separated
- 2 teaspoons of coriander seeds
- 1 tablespoon of olive oil
- 1 yellow onion, chopped
- Salt and black pepper to the taste
- A pinch of red pepper, crushed
- 1 small ginger piece, chopped
- 1 garlic clove, minced
- 28 ounces of canned tomatoes, pureed

Directions:

1. Heat a medium-hot pan that matches the oil with your Air Fryer, add the onions, salt, pepper, and red pepper, combine and cook for seven minutes.

2. Add the ginger, garlic, cilantro, tomatoes and broccoli, stir, add to the Air Fryer and cook at 360 degrees F for 12 minutes.

3. Break and serve in pots.

75.Collard Greens and Bacon

Total time: 22 min

Prep time: 7 min

Cook time: 15 min

Yield: 4 servings

Ingredients:

- 1-pound collard greens
- 3 bacon strips, chopped
- ¼ cup cherry tomatoes halved
- 1 tablespoon of apple cider vinegar
- 2 tablespoons of chicken stock
- Salt and black pepper to the taste

Directions:

1. Heat a medium-pressure saucepan, add the bacon, stir and cook for 1-2 minutes.
2. Add the tomatoes, collard greens, vinegar, stock, salt and pepper, blend, add to the Air Fryer and cook at 320 degrees F for 10 minutes.
3. Divide and feed between bowls.

76.Sesame Mustard Greens

Total time: 22 min

Prep time: 7 min

Cook time: 15 min

Yield: 4 servings

Ingredients:

- 2 garlic cloves, minced
- 1-pound of mustard greens, torn
- 1 tablespoon of olive oil
- ½ cup yellow onion, sliced
- Salt and black pepper to the taste

- 3 tablespoons of veggie stock
- ¼ teaspoon of dark sesame oil

Directions:

1. Heat a medium-hot saucepan that suits the grease of your Air Fryer, add the onions, blend and brown for 5 minutes.
2. Add the garlic, stock, onions, salt, and pepper, stir, add to the Air Fryer, and cook at 350 degrees F for 6 minutes.
3. Tie the sesame oil together, swirl to coat, break and serve in cups.

77.Radish Hash

Total time: 18 min

Prep time: 5 min

Cook time. 10 min

Yield: 4 servings

Ingredients:

- ½ teaspoon of onion powder
- 1-pound radishes, sliced
- ½ teaspoon of garlic powder
- Salt and black pepper to the taste
- 4 eggs
- 1/3 cup of parmesan, grated

Directions:

1. In a bowl of salt, pepper, onion and garlic powder, eggs, and parmesan cheese, combine the radishes, then whisk well.
2. Shift the radishes into a fridge-friendly saucepan and simmer at 350° F for 7 minutes.
3. Divide the hash into bowls and serve.

78.Cod Pie with Palmit

Preparation Time: 15 Minutes

Cooking Time: 30 Minutes

Servings: 4-6

Ingredients:

- 2 ¼ lb cod
- 4 ½ lb of natural heart previously grated and cooked
- 12 eggs
- 1 ½ cup olive oil
- 7 oz. of olives
- Tomato Chopped garlic, paprika and sliced onion
- Green seasoning

Directions:

1. In a frying pan, cook the cod and, after cooking, destroy it.

2. Drain the heart of the palm well on the reservation.

3. Along with tomatoes, garlic, paprika, ginger, green seasoning and half of the pitted olives, sauté the cod and palm hearts in olive oil for 20 minutes.

4. Pour 6 eggs into the sample and stir for 5 minutes.

5. Grease the olive oil trays and place the mixture into them.

6. Beat the rest of the eggs and spill over the top evenly.

7. Add tomatoes and olives to garnish.

8. Bake for 40 minutes in the air-fryer at 3800F.

79.Simple and Yummy Cod
Preparation Time: 10 Minutes

Cooking Time: 15 Minutes

Servings: 4-6

Ingredients:

- 2 ¼ lb of desalted cod
- 1 ½ lb of boiled and squeezed potatoes
- 1 can of sour cream
- 2 large onions, sliced

- 1 pot of pitted olive
- ½ cup of olive oil
- Butter for greasing

Directions:

1. In the oil, marinate the onions until they wilt.

2. Give the cod a further 5 minutes to sauté.

3. Add the sour cream and potato and stir for another 5 minutes.

4. Turn the heat off and add some more oil.

5. Place the cod in a refractory greased butter and pass the margarine over it again to render it golden.

6. Bake at 4000F for about 20 minutes or until golden brown in an air fryer.

7. It's fast and delicious to serve with rice.

80.Roasted Tilapia Fillet
Preparation Time: 10 Minutes

Cooking Time: 15 Minutes

Servings: 4-6

Ingredients:

- 2 ¼ lb tilapia fillet
- ½ lemon juice
- 4 sliced tomatoes
- 4 sliced onions
- ½ cup chopped black olives
- 1 pound of boiled potatoes
- 1 tbsp. butter ½ cup sour cream tea
- ½ lb grated mozzarella Olive oil Salt

Directions:

1. With lemon and salt, season the fillets.

2. Place a sheet of onions and tomatoes on an ovenproof tray. On top of the layers, position the fillets.

3. Marinade with another layer of tomato and onion, then the olives and drizzle with the olive oil.

4. Bake in an air-fryer for 15 minutes at 3600F.

5. Squeeze the potatoes in another bowl.

6. Melt the butter in a saucepan. Put the cream with both the potatoes.

7. Place this puree on top of the fillets, then place the mozzarella on top of them.

8. Bake for another 5 minutes in an air fryer at 3600F and serve.

81. Cod 7-Mares
Preparation Time: 10 Minutes

Cooking Time: 15 Minutes

Servings: 4-6

Ingredients:

- 1 lb cod in French fries
- 4 large potatoes, peeled and diced
- 1 can of cream without serum
- 1 cup of coffee with coconut milk
- 3 ½ oz. of mozzarella cheese in strips
- 3 ½ oz. cheese in pieces
- 100 g3 ½ oz. grated Parmesan cheese
- Aromatic herbs and salt to taste.
- 1 tbsp. of curry
- Salt to taste

Directions:

1. Cook and set aside the peeled and diced potatoes.

2. Remove the salt from the cod (leave it overnight in the water and at least change the water

3 times to have the salt erased). 3. Place the potatoes in a glass jar and cook in the microwave for 5 minutes. Set aside.

4. The cream, coconut milk, curry, mozzarella cheese, and herbs are mixed in a bowl. Mounting Up

5. Top a layer of boiled potatoes on a pan, put the cod fries on top, and pour the sauce on top.

6. Season to taste with salt.

7. Sprinkle with Parmesan cheese and cook in an air fryer at 3600F for 7 minutes.

8. Toss the chives over the top when done, and immediately serve.

82.Roasted Hake with Coconut Milk
Preparation Time: 10 Minutes

Cooking Time: 30 Minutes

Servings: 2

Ingredients:

- 2 ¼ lb hake fillet
- ½ lb sliced mozzarella
- 1 can of sour cream
- 1 bottle of coconut milk
- 1 onion
- 1 tomato
- Salt and black pepper to taste.
- Lemon juice

Directions:

1. With salt, pepper and lemon, season the fillets.

2. Let them stand for ten minutes.

3. Arrange the fillets and put each one in the center of the mozzarella slices and roll it up like a fillet.

4. The fillets were rolled up after all.

5. Just get a tray.

6. Place on top of the tomato and onion slices (sliced).

7. Attach the sour cream and coconut milk mixture to the top.

8. Bake for 20 minutes inside an air-fryer at 4000, coated with aluminum foil.

9. Then, to finish baking, remove it.

83.Air fryer Catfish
Preparation Time: 15 Minutes

Cooking Time: 1 Hour

Servings: 2-4

Ingredients:

- 3 pounds sliced dogfish
- 1 pound boiled and sliced potatoes
- 1 package of onion cream
- 3 tomatoes cut into slices
- 3 bell peppers cut into slices
- 3 onions cut into slices
- Olive oil
- 2 garlic cloves, crushed
- Salt to taste
- 1 lemon juice

Directions:

1. With garlic, salt and ginger, season the fish slices and set them aside.

2. Place the potatoes on a baking sheet to get the slices and drizzle with plenty of oil, forming a kind of bed.

3. On the potatoes, spread half of the onion cream.

4. Lay on top of the slices.

5. Place on top of the tomato, bell pepper and onion, spread well and cover the slices. Drizzle with olive oil again, and then pour on top of the rest of the onion cream.

6. Heat the air fryer at 3600F for about 15 minutes and then bake for 1 hour.

84.Squid to the Milanese

Preparation Time: 5 Minutes

Cooking Time: 15 Minutes

Servings: 4-6

Ingredients:

- 2 ¼ lb clean squid
- Salt, pepper and oregano to taste.
- 3 beaten eggs
- 1 cup of wheat flour
- 1 cup breadcrumbs
- 1 cup chopped green chives

Directions:

1. Season the squid with salt, pepper and oregano, after washing and cutting into rings.

2. Put the squid over the beaten eggs, then mix the breadcrumbs with the wheat flour.

3. Fry for 10 minutes in the air-fryer at 4000F. 4. Green onions are sprinkled.

85.Portugal Codfish with Cream

Preparation Time: 10 Minutes

Cooking Time: 15 Minutes

Servings: 2-4

Ingredients:

- 2 ¼ lbs of cod
- 1 chopped onion
- 2 cloves of garlic
- 4 medium potatoes
- 1 leek stalk (Portugal leek)

- 2 cups of cream
- 1 egg Parmesan
- Coriander (optional)
- Olive oil
- Black olives

Directions:

1. Soak the cod in water for approximately 24 hours until the salt is to your taste.

2. Put the oil and brown the garlic, the onion and the leek in a frying pan, then place the cod and let it brown.

3. Take the diced potatoes and cook them separately.

4. Then, with the golden cod, bring the potatoes together. Then put the cilantro along with the cream or sour cream to your liking. Integrate everything.

5. Spread a little Parmesan on top, beat 1 whole egg and sprinkle the cod and marinade with black olives.

6. Place it at 3600F for 30 minutes in an air fryer or until it turns into a crispy cone.

7. Serve with a lovely salad of lettuce, nothing more.

86.Roasted Salmon with Provencal

Preparation Time: 10 Minutes

Cooking Time: 20 Minutes

Servings: 2

Ingredients:

- 4 slices of fresh salmon basil thyme
- Rosemary oregano salt and pepper olive oil
- 4 tablespoons of butter
- ½ lemon juice

Directions:

1. On a hot plate, place the salmon slices and sprinkle with the 4 herbs.

2. Then add salt, pepper and a couple of drops of olive oil to taste.

3. Bake for 15 minutes at 4000F in an air fryer (check every 5 minutes).

4. Serve with potatoes, herbal butter and a new salad.

5. Until it's creamy, whip the butter.

6. Add the same lemon juice and the herbs described previously.

87.Breaded Fish with Tartar Sauce

Preparation Time: 15 Minutes

Cooking Time: 20 Minutes

Servings: 2-4

Ingredients:

- 1 lb of hake fillet
- 4 garlic cloves, crushed
- Juice of 2 lemons
- Salt and black pepper
- Beaten eggs
- Wheat flour
- Vegetable oil for frying

Sauce:

- 3 oz. green olives
- 3 tbsp. chopped onion
- 1 garlic clove, crushed
- Parsley and chives
- 5 tbsp. soy sauce
- ½ can of cream
- 3 tbsp. of dijon mustard
- 1 tbsp. of tomato sauce
- 4 tbsp. mayonnaise

Tartar sauce:

- ½ lb chopped pickles

Directions:

1. Season the fillets with salt, pepper, garlic, and lemon juice, let them taste for at least 30 minutes.

2. Pass the wheat, egg and wheat again.

3. Fry them in the air fryer at 4000F for 25 minutes.

4. Mix all the ingredients in a bowl. 5. Serve with the fillets.

88.Milanese Fish Fillet

Preparation Time: 10 Minutes

Cooking Time: 30 Minutes

Servings: 2-3

Ingredients:

- 1 lb of fish fillet of your choice
- Salt
- 2 garlic cloves, crushed
- 3 eggs Wheat flour
- Oil for frying

Directions:

1. Wash and season the fish fillets with garlic and salt.

2. If you want, you can add the juice of a lemon.

3. Beat the egg whites until stiff and add the egg yolks.

4. Pass the fish fillets, one at a time, in the wheat flour and then pass them over the beaten eggs in the snow.

5. Fry in the air fryer at 4000F for 25 minutes or until they are golden brown.

89.Sole with White Wine

Preparation Time: 10 Minutes

Cooking Time: 35 Minutes

Servings: 4-6

Ingredients:

- 3 lbs of sole fillets
- 5 ¼ oz. of butter
- 1 glass of white wine
- Wheat flour
- Salt black pepper thyme

Directions:

1. Season the fillet with both the wheat flour and pass it on.

2. For 20 minutes or until brown, put in an air fryer at 4000F. In a preheated clay pan, reserve this fish.

3. In the butter, toast a tablespoon of flour.

4. Add the wine to taste, with salt, pepper and thyme. Let everything cook for another three minutes, stirring constantly. Pour the sole over and eat.

90.Golden Fish with Shrimps

Preparation Time: 10 Minutes

Cooking Time: 30 Minutes

Servings: 2-3

Ingredients:

- 1 large golden fish
- 1 lb of shrimp onion
- tomato
- Pepper
- lemon
- olive oil
- Butter
- green smell parsley

Directions:

1. Clean the complete golden and season with lemon, black pepper to taste and salt, the same with the prawns.

2. Leave for 1 hour after seasoning.

3. Place the fish on this plate, add the shrimp to the fish's belly, and tie it with a line. Line a plate with aluminum foil and grease with butter.

4. On top of the gold, put the onion rings, tomatoes and peppers and the green odor with the parsley and use it with plenty of oil.

5. Cover the tray with aluminum foil and bake for 35 minutes at 4000F in the air fryer.

6. With white rice, serve.

91.Stroganoff Cod

Preparation Time: 5 Minutes

Cooking Time: 35 Minutes

Servings: 4-6

Ingredients:

- 1 lb of cod
- 3 tbsp. olive oil
- 2 garlic cloves, minced
- 2 ¼ lb of chopped onion
- 4 ½ lb of skinless tomatoes
- Salt to taste
- ½ cup of brandy
- Oregano, rosemary and black pepper to taste.
- 1 package of chopped green aroma
- 1 cup grated cheese
- 2 ¼ lb of fresh mushrooms cut into chips
- 1 can of sour cream
- 1 large golden fish
- 1 lb of shrimp onion tomato
- Pepper lemon olive oil
- Butter green smell parsley

Directions:

1. Soak the cod in water the day before, boil and crumble all the meat. Reserve. Reserve.

2. In olive oil, saute the onion and garlic. Add the tomatoes that have been chopped and boil until separated. Remove. Remove!

3. Season with salt, oregano, rosemary and black pepper. Blend with the cod and apply the brandy. Add the mushrooms and the green odor.

4. Put it in an air-fryer for 10 minutes at 3200. Taking the fryer out of the air; add the grated cheese and sour cream.

5. Mix well with white rice and serve.

92.Cod Balls

Preparation Time: 10 Minutes

Cooking Time: 15 Minutes

Servings: 2-4

Ingredients:

- ½ lb salted and grated cod
- 3 cups boiled and squeezed potatoes
- 1 tbsp. of wheat flour
- Salt and black pepper to taste
- 3 eggs
- 2 tbsp. chopped green aroma

Directions:

1. In a bowl, mix all the ingredients well.

2. Form the balls with your hands.

3. Fry in the air fryer at 4000F for 30 minutes or until golden brown.

93.Lobster Bang Bang

Preparation Time: 15 Minutes

Cooking Time: 20 Minutes

Servings: 4

Ingredients:

- 1 cup cornstarch
- ¼ teaspoon Sriracha powder
- ¼ cup mayonnaise
- ¼ cup sweet chili sauce
- 4 lbs Lobsters

Directions:

1. In a big bowl, combine corn-starch and Sriracha powder.

2. Dredge lobsters with this mixture.

3. Place lobsters in the air fryer.

4. Choose an air fry setting.

5. Cook at 400 degrees F for 7 minutes per side.

6. Mix the mayo and chili sauce.

7. Serve shrimp with sauce.

94.Honey Glazed Salmon

Preparation Time: 10 Minutes

Cooking Time: 35 Minutes

Servings: 1

Ingredients:

- ¼ cup soy sauce
- ½ cup honey

- 1 tablespoon lemon juice
- 1 oz. orange juice
- 1 tablespoon brown sugar
- 1 teaspoon olive oil
- 1 tablespoon red wine vinegar
- 1 scallion, chopped
- 1 clove garlic, minced
- Salt and pepper to taste
- 1 salmon fillet

Directions:

1. Mix all the ingredients except salt, pepper and salmon.

2. Place mixture in a pan over medium heat.

3. Bring to a boil.

4. Reduce heat.

5. Simmer for 15 minutes.

6. Turn off heat and transfer sauce to a bowl.

7. Sprinkle salt and pepper on both sides of the salmon.

8. Add salmon to the air fryer.

9. Select grill function.

95.Crispy Fish Fillet

Preparation Time: 10 Minutes

Cooking Time: 30 Minutes

Servings: 2

Ingredients:

- 2 cod fillets
- 1 teaspoon Old Bay seasoning
- Salt and pepper to taste
- ½ cup all-purpose flour

- 1 egg, beaten
- 2 cups breadcrumbs

Directions:

1. Sprinkle both sides of cod with Old Bay seasoning, salt and pepper.

2. Coat with flour, dip in egg and dredge with breadcrumbs.

3. Add fish to the air fryer.

4. Select air fry setting.

5. Cook at 400 degrees F for 5 to 6 minutes per side.

96.Garlic Butter Lobster Tails

Preparation Time: 10 Minutes

Cooking Time: 15 Minutes

Servings: 2

Ingredients:

- 2 lobster tails
- 2 cloves garlic, minced
- 2 tablespoons butter
- 1 teaspoon lemon juice
- 1 teaspoon chopped chives
- Salt to taste

Directions:

1. Butterfly the lobster tails.

2. Place the meat on top of the shell.

3. Mix the remaining ingredients in a bowl.

4. Add lobster tails inside the air fryer.

5. Set it to air fry.

6. Spread garlic butter on the meat.

7. Cook at 380 degrees F for 5 minutes.

8. Spread more butter on top.

9. Cook for another 2 to 3 minutes.

97.Pesto Fish

Preparation Time: 10 Minutes

Cooking Time: 15 Minutes

Servings: 4

Ingredients:

- 1 tablespoon olive oil
- 4 fish fillets
- Salt and pepper to taste
- 1 cup olive oil
- 3 cloves garlic
- 1 ½ cups fresh basil leaves
- 2 tablespoons Parmesan cheese, grated
- 3 tablespoons pine nuts

Directions:

1. Drizzle olive oil over fish fillets and season with salt and pepper.

2. Add remaining ingredients to a food processor.

3. Pulse until smooth.

4. Transfer pesto to a bowl and set aside.

5. Add fish to the air fryer.

6. Select grill setting.

7. Cook at 320 degrees F for 5 minutes per side.

8. Spread pesto on top of the fish before serving.

98.Mozzarella Spinach Quiche

Prep time: 10 min

Cook time: 45 min

Yield: 6 servings

Ingredients:

- 4 eggs
- 10 oz. frozen spinach, thawed
- 1/2 cup mozzarella cheese, shredded
- 1/4 cup parmesan cheese, grated
- 8 oz. mushrooms, sliced
- 2 oz. feta cheese, crumbled
- 1 cup almond milk
- 1 garlic clove, minced
- Pepper
- Salt

Directions:

27. Spray a pie dish with cooking spray and set it aside.
28. Insert wire rack in rack position 6. Select bake, set temperature 350 f, timer for 45 minutes. Press start to preheat the oven.
29. Spray medium pan with cooking spray and heat over medium heat.
30. Add garlic, mushrooms, pepper, and salt in a pan and sauté for 5 minutes.
31. Add spinach to the pie dish, then add sautéed mushroom on top of spinach.
32. Sprinkle feta cheese over spinach and mushroom.
33. In a bowl, whisk eggs, parmesan cheese, and almond milk.
34. Pour egg mixture over spinach and mushroom, then sprinkle shredded mozzarella cheese and bake for 45 minutes.
35. Sliced and serve.

99.Cheesy Zucchini Quiche

Total time: 1 hour 10 min

Prep time: 10 min

Cook time: 60 min

Yield: 8 servings

Ingredients:

- 2 eggs
- 2 cups cheddar cheese, shredded
- 1 1/2 cup almond milk
- Pepper
- Salt
- 2 lbs. zucchini, sliced

Directions:

1. Set aside and oil the quiche pan with cooking oil.
2. Wire rack insertion at rack position 6. Pick bake, set temperature to 375 f, 60-minute timer. To preheat the oven, press start.
3. With pepper and salt, season the zucchini and set aside for 30 minutes.
4. Mix the almond milk, spice, and salt with the eggs in a big cup.
5. Stir well and Mix sliced cheddar cheese.
6. Arrange slices of zucchini in a plate of quiche.
7. Pour the combination of eggs over the slices of zucchini and scatter with shredded cheese. For 60 minutes, roast.
8. Enjoy and serve.

100.Healthy Asparagus Quiche

Total time: 1 hour 10 min

Prep time: 10 min

Cook time: 60 min

Yield: 6 servings

Ingredients:

- 5 eggs, beaten
- 1 cup almond milk

- 15 asparagus spears, cut ends then cut asparagus in half
- 1 cup Swiss cheese, shredded
- 1/4 tsp. thyme
- 1/4 tsp. white pepper
- 1/4 tsp. salt

Directions:

Grease quiche pan with cooking spray and set aside.

Insert wire rack in rack position 6. Select bake, set temperature 350 f, timer for 60 minutes. Press start to preheat the oven.

In a bowl, whisk together eggs, thyme, white pepper, almond milk, and salt.

Arrange asparagus in quiche pan, then pour egg mixture over asparagus. Sprinkle with shredded cheese.

Bake for 60 minutes.

Sliced and serve.

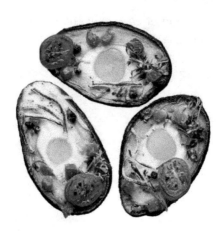

Conclusion

Before you know how to use an Air Fryer, you need to make some plans before using it and take some steps accordingly. Such as getting an amazing recipe book to cook your food using an air fryer. This book will surely help you with that as it has covered a delicious range of air fryer recipes.

CPSIA information can be obtained
at www.ICGtesting.com
Printed in the USA
BVHW050157060321
601818BV00006B/743

9 781802 163056